T0276868

Encyclopedia of Diabetes: Prevention and Treatment of Type 2 Diabetes

Volume 13

Encyclopedia of Diabetes: Prevention and Treatment of Type 2 Diabetes
Volume 13

Edited by **Rex Slavin, Windy Wise and Roy Marcus Cohn**

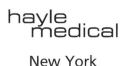

New York

Published by Hayle Medical,
30 West, 37th Street, Suite 612,
New York, NY 10018, USA
www.haylemedical.com

Encyclopedia of Diabetes: Prevention and Treatment of Type 2 Diabetes
Volume 13
Edited by Rex Slavin, Windy Wise and Roy Marcus Cohn

© 2015 Hayle Medical

International Standard Book Number: 978-1-63241-155-6 (Hardback)

This book contains information obtained from authentic and highly regarded sources. Copyright for all individual chapters remain with the respective authors as indicated. A wide variety of references are listed. Permission and sources are indicated; for detailed attributions, please refer to the permissions page. Reasonable efforts have been made to publish reliable data and information, but the authors, editors and publisher cannot assume any responsibility for the validity of all materials or the consequences of their use.

The publisher's policy is to use permanent paper from mills that operate a sustainable forestry policy. Furthermore, the publisher ensures that the text paper and cover boards used have met acceptable environmental accreditation standards.

Trademark Notice: Registered trademark of products or corporate names are used only for explanation and identification without intent to infringe.

Printed in the United States of America.

Contents

Permissions

List of Contributors

Preface

The purpose of the book is to provide a glimpse into the dynamics and to present opinions and studies of some of the scientists engaged in the development of new ideas in the field from very different standpoints. This book will prove useful to students and researchers owing to its high content quality.

Type-2 Diabetes is a severe health problem worldwide. Patients with this disease have 2-4 times greater risk of renal and cardiovascular complications, mortality and morbidity. Comprehending the etiology of the onset and advancement of this disease is crucial to avoid its complications and delay the progress. This book covers important topics under treatments and prevention. The prevention and treatments contains detailed accounts regarding bariatric surgery, insulin therapy, pharmacological and non-pharmacological treatments. The aim of this book is to provide the readers with helpful knowledge regarding the field and assist clinicians and researchers.

At the end, I would like to appreciate all the efforts made by the authors in completing their chapters professionally. I express my deepest gratitude to all of them for contributing to this book by sharing their valuable works. A special thanks to my family and friends for their constant support in this journey.

Editor

Prevention and Treatments

Screening for Diabetes in Family Practice: A Case Study in Ontario, Canada

Gina Agarwal

Additional information is available at the end of the chapter

1. Introduction

1.1. Prevalence and Incidence of Diabetes in Ontario, Canada

The scale of the problem of diabetes in family practice is described with respect to prevalence and incidence in family medicine.

Type 2 diabetes (T2DM) and prediabetes [impaired fasting glucose (IFG); impaired glucose tolerance (IGT); and / or both IFG and IGT] are common metabolic disturbances in Canada and worldwide, having long been recognized to be reaching close to epidemic proportions [1]. Indeed, the global prevalence of diabetes in 2011 was 8.3% [2]. According to the National Diabetes Surveillance System, in 2009, over 2 million Canadians were estimated to have T2DM; a prevalence of T2DM 6.4% [3]. As many as one in six people over the age of 65 years are currently estimated to have diabetes [4]. Adults from lower income groups are twice as likely to have diabetes as those in the highest income groups [4]. Estimates suggest that over 5 million Canadians had prediabetes in 2004; a prevalence of 23% for ages 40 to 74 years [5]. The prevalence of IFG is more frequent in women but both IFG and IGT increase in prevalence with age [6].

2. Predicted increase in numbers of people with diabetes

Alarmingly, diabetes prevalence is expected to increase significantly; this will be described in detail with respect to the effect on the primary care system.

The global prevalence for diabetes is predicted to be 9.9% in 2030, an increase of approximately 20% in 20 years [2]. Indeed, over time, the prevalence of Type 2 Diabetes (T2DM)

in Ontario has increased at a much faster rate than anticipated. Adult diabetes prevalence in Ontario rose by 80%, from 5% in 1995, to 9% in 2005[6], thereby exceeding the global prevalence increase of T2DM of 6.4% projected for 2030 [7]. Following that, over a 6 year period, a 31% increase in yearly incidence occurred in Canada, from 6.6 per 1,000 in 1997 to 8.2 per 1,000 in 2003 [7]. The diabetes epidemic is not restricted to Canada, as 1 in 10 adults in the USA now have diabetes [8].

Increasing numbers of people with diabetes will result in more healthcare resources being utilised [5,6,7]. Current estimates suggest that people with diabetes use five-times as many health resources as those without [9]. Therefore, developing and testing effective strategies to increase detection of diabetes in the community is an important primary care and population health issue. Furthermore, up to one third of the people with diabetes are estimated to be undiagnosed [8,10] and may be developing diabetes-related complications which may also remain undiagnosed. Not only will the utilisation of healthcare resources be restricted to diabetes-related micro and macro vascular diseases, but other conditions as well. People with diabetes or dysglycemia are at over a twofold risk of developing cardiovascular disease compared to diabetes-free individuals [11,12,13]. These factors point to the seriousness of the diabetes epidemic and its potential impact.

3. Progression of prediabetes to diabetes

The speed at which prediabetes progresses to diabetes has serious implications for adequate healthcare. The scale of this will be discussed in depth.

Individuals with prediabetes are estimated to progress to type 2 diabetes at a rate of 10-12% per year; in total up to as much as 70% will progress [14-16]. Furthermore, individuals with both IFG and IGT develop type 2 diabetes at approximately twice the rate as those who have only one of these impairments [17]. The speed at which prediabetes progresses to diabetes has serious implications for adequate healthcare provision to the adult Canadian population aged 40 and over (which represented approximately 50% of the Canadian population in the 2006 census) [18].

Since diabetes is a multi-system metabolic chronic disorder, it causes complications that affect many organs including eyes, nerves and kidneys as well as other health related consequences. Specific complications of diabetes include macrovascular (i.e. coronary artery disease), and microvascular (i.e. renal damage, nerve damage and retinal damage) [19]. Treatment for diabetes consists of dietary and lifestyle changes, oral medication and injected insulin [19]. The healthcare system will be stretched having to care for an epidemic of people with diabetic complications.

However, pharmacological and lifestyle interventions could prevent or delay T2DM and thus decrease morbidity and mortality associated with its complications if individuals at risk of developing diabetes are detected early [20]. Unfortunately, only 49% of Canadians over 40 years old report ever having a diabetes screening blood test sometime during their life [21] and much diabetes and prediabetes remains undiagnosed [10]. Future treatment costs could possibly be avoided by increasing prevention and screening efforts.

4. Diagnosis of diabetes

This section will outline the many tests possible and the best choices for family physicians.

Prediabetes and diabetes can be diagnosed with inexpensive fasting blood tests [either a fasting plasma glucose (FPG) level or a 75-gram oral glucose tolerance test (OGTT). The WHO 2006 diagnostic criteria provide the appropriate cut-off points for blood tests interpretation (see Table 1) [22]. The FPG test is commonly used by Canadian physicians to identify those with prediabetes and diabetes [21].

Measurement of only a FPG misses 15% or more of people with IGT [23,24]; but, using the diagnostic criteria for IFG identifies a different and smaller group of people compared to using criteria for IGT [25,26]. Although the oral glucose tolerance test (OGTT) is the diagnostic gold standard, cost and impracticality limit its use as a screening test (overnight fasting and a 2-hour laboratory wait are required). In addition glycosylated hemoglobin or A1c is already being used as a diagnostic test by many physicians. The American Diabetes Association in 2010 recommended that A1c could be used as a screening test in non-pregnant individuals, and those without chronic kidney, liver or blood disorders which can all affect the hemoglobin levels [27]. Their recommendations state that an A1c of 6.5% (47 mmol/mol) or higher indicates diabetes and an A1c of 5.7% - 6.4% (39 - 46 mmol/mol) is indicative of prediabetes.

The Canadian Diabetes Association has also followed suit and recommended that A1c be used as a screening tool with the same limitations, and diagnostic for diabetes above 6.5%, however two separate readings (two of a combination of A1c or FPG) are required for diagnosis [28]. Increasingly, there is debate concerning the use of other laboratory tests since although the OGTT is the gold standard it may not be used frequently (Ontario data shows that less than 1% of people underwent an OGTT between 1995 and 2005) [29]. An increasing number of individuals without documented diabetes in Ontario have been tested using the A1c [1]. Additionally, many Ontarians receive serum blood glucose testing, which is either random or fasting (80% of women and 66% of men) [30].

	Fasting Plasma Glucose (mmol/l)	2 hour Post 75g Glucose Load (mmol/l)
T2DM	≥7.0	≥11.1
Isolated IGT	<6.1	7.8-11.0
Isolated IFG	6.1 – 6.9	<7.8
IGT and IFG	6.1 – 6.9	7.8-11.0
Normal	<6.1	<7.8

Table 1. Diagnostic Criteria for Diabetes and Prediabetes [22,31,32]

5. Screening for diabetes

The use of risk assessment tools in general practice will be discussed with reference to the literature.

Though T2DM can often remain undiagnosed and asymptomatic in its early stages [33], once diagnosed, it can be treated with lifestyle modification and medication, and some elements of the disease process may be reversible [14,16,34]. In light of this, early T2DM detection may be beneficial to both patients and society [35]. Screening may also detect people at high risk of developing diabetes; and thereby, determine the likelihood that a person may have a positive diagnosis of diabetes.

Screening for diabetes can be approached in 3 different ways; opportunistic, risk-based or universal. Opportunistic screening occurs where a health care practitioner will screen as part of routine medical care, whether this is part of a physical examination or other arising medical interaction [36]. Risk-based screening focuses on screening individuals at high risk of developing diabetes due to a health related trait that they have, such as obesity, age, positive family history [37]. Universal screening would screen everyone irrespective of characteristics [37] or just use age and gender criteria for screening.

Since the OGTT is the gold standard, including it in any screening program for diabetes and prediabetes may therefore be an important strategy [37], though impractical for universal screening. The challenge is how to improve the overall accuracy of diabetes screening, and to incorporate OGTT at a reasonable cost, by incorporating it as part of a multi-stage screening process. This two-step approach has already been tested and proven in Finland, and is now being implemented across many European countries as an emerging best practice. Literature demonstrates that non-laboratory based questionnaires (e.g. the FINRISK) to pre-identify individuals at risk of T2DM and prediabetes can be successful [38,39]. Screening questionnaires have similar diagnostic accuracy to laboratory screening tests and are inexpensive, simple to use and can also be used as educational tools for patients undergoing screening [38,39,40]. They can be used in conjunction with laboratory testing for universal screening.

An effectively screened population will have diabetes diagnosed 5–6 years earlier than a population without an organized screening program [41], offering opportunies for delaying diabetes and related complications [16]. The current screening tests of repeated serum glucose measurements are too costly and inconvenient to be offered at a population level in the form of a screening program. Furthermore, the organization of primary care in Canada is poorly designed to cope with the initiation and management of comprehensive diabetes screening for everyone over 40 years of age [36]. Existing diabetes prevention and lifestyle programs, designed for research and not community application, have unrealistic program costs, since they require all participants to have OGTTs [42,43]. However, sequential and selective screening of high-risk groups could increase efficiency [44] and reduce workload and screening costs for the healthcare system by reducing the number of individuals requiring a 'gold standard' diagnostic test, as compared to universal screening [45,46].

6. Role of family practitioners

This chapter will clarify what the best method of screening is for family physicians by examining the evidence and provide recommendations for current practice.

In light of the evidence for early treatment of diabetes, in the Canadian Diabetes Association (CDA) clinical practice guidelines [31,32], the recommendations are clear that individuals at high risk for developing diabetes should be screened to determine their dysglycemic status, in an attempt to be able to recommend changes to lifestyle which may prevent or delay the onset of diabetes. 'High risk' is defined as a person whose first degree relatives have diabetes, and/or who have other diabetes risk factors such as ethnic origin, obesity and dyslipidemia, and who have a FPG of 5.7-6.9 mmol/L. Though not explicitly stated, the implementation of this screening recommendation is the responsibility of family doctors, since traditionally they are the first point of access to health care in Canada. Family doctors usually have the opportunity to detect diabetes in their patients at annual health checks as long as the patient has a physical exam. However, at least 15% of the Canadian population does not have a family doctor and will not receive a physical examination [47]. Family doctors are a scarce resource and may not be able to initiate successful screening programs for all their patients. Indeed, evidence shows that they may be too busy [33], or resources too scarce to implement comprehensive screening either opportunistically or targeted, or to provide appropriate follow up to identified individuals. Therefore, opportunistic screening in this way may not be the best approach to effectively identify the individuals with diabetes. Other strategies may be more appropriate, but few have been tested or rigorously evaluated in family practice.

Rather than a universal screening program of everybody over the age of 40 years, selective screening of subgroups at high risk of having the disease may reduce the workload and the cost to the healthcare system by reducing the number of individuals who need a diagnostic test [48], while still identifying the vast majority of new cases. Involving patients themselves in the decision to attend screening may also lessen the burden on family physicians, since a consultation initiated for risk assessment alone, is likely to be more focused than one initiated for other reasons [49]. Taking into account these issues, a program utilising this philosophy, the Community Health Awareness of Diabetes program, was developed and piloted in Ontario. CHAD assessed risk of diabetes in the over 40 year old population using the Finnish Diabetes Risk Score [38] (for impaired glucose tolerance detection), the Cambridge Diabetes Risk Score [50] (for undiagnosed diabetes), fasting capillary blood glucose and a glycosylated hemoglobin level. Individuals were invited by their family doctors, for 'diabetes awareness and risk assessment' sessions delivered by specially trained community peers, in a network of local community pharmacies.

There were 588 participants in CHAD; of these, the majority that had received invitation letters were seniors and were females; 526 did not have pre-existing diabetes; and 16% of participants were identified as being at high risk for diabetes [51]. Those at high risk of diabetes had significantly more modifiable risk factors, including higher fat, fast food and salt intake, and higher systolic blood pressure. Satisfaction with the program was high. An audit of 1030 medical charts of individuals eligible to attend the CHAD program, from 28 family doctors' practices in Grimsby, Ontario. Of these, 387 charts were of patients who had attended the CHAD program and 643 charts were of individuals who did not attend the program but who met the program eligibility criteria. Overall, the difference between the rates of diabetes diagnosis before-and-after the program was not statistically different. The difference in rate of diabetes diagnosis annually in the attendee group was 20 per 1000 and in the non-attendee group was -2 (to be interpreted as 0) per 1000. In the community, the annual rate of new diabetes diagnosis was 27 per 1000 (95% CI = 17.90 – 39.00) in the year before the introduction of the CHAD program, and 45 per 1000 (95% CI = 33.00 – 59.80) in the year after.

The attendee and non-attendee groups were significantly different demographically in that the CHAD attendees were more likely to be female, retried and older than the random sample of eligible patients drawn from the same practices. Multi-level regression modeling showed that attending CHAD did seem to have a positive effect on whether diabetes was diagnosed; however, this effect was lessened both in statistical significance and magnitude when taking in to account the physician effect (clustering), patient gender, patient employment status and patient age. If found to be effective in both case detection and cost, a targeted community diabetes screening program should be recommended to Canadian Health Policy makers. Current literature shows that screening is more cost effective in hypertensive and obese groups and the costs of screening are offset in many groups by lower treatment costs [52].

7. Conclusions

The debate for or against screening and even the method of screening in the community therefore has not been fully resolved in Canada. Currently, though the Canadian Diabetes Association recommends screening all individuals over the age of 40 [31,32], the Canadian Task Force on Preventive Health Care (CTFPHC) recommends screening only for adults with hypertension or hyperlipidemia [46]. Both guidelines are under frequent review and revision. For now, health policy makers will need to assess their own communities' needs, which may vary based on the population mix, and assess whether or not local programs for screening (whether targeted or universal) could be initiated; an example of this is the Aboriginal Diabetes Initiative [53]. Through this program, targeting the Aboriginal population increased regular screening for early diagnosis using population-based and opportunistic screening methods is supported, with the use of mobile detection programs. It is possible that diabetes screening could be increased in communities predicted by population-based algorithms to have high rates of undiagnosed diabetes [54]. Researchers have used population based data (national registries and other such data) and developed and validated an algorithm to estimate the number of individuals who will develop diabetes over a 9-year period [54]. This algorithm could be applied to existing provincial data to decide where to focus diabetes screening strategies for greatest effect.

Those reading this chapter from other countries must evaluate the need for screening for diabetes or at the very least, risk-assessment for diabetes, in the primary care setting, which is the natural setting for such activities. Given the epidemic of diabetes worldwide, it is likely that many other countries will be able to use the case study example posed here, as a way of evaluating the need to screen in primary care or family medicine situations elsewhere.

Author details

Gina Agarwal

Department of Family Medicine, McMaster University, Canada

References

[1] Health Canada (1999) Diabetes in Canada: National Statistics and Opportunities for Improved Surveillance, Prevention, and Control. Catalogue No. H49-121/1999. Ottawa: Laboratory Centre for Disease Control, Bureau of Cardio-Respiratory Diseases and Diabetes.

[2] IDF 5th Diabetes Atlas: The Global Burden of Diabetes. http://www.idf.org/diabete-satlas/5e/the-global-burden accessed 12th December 2012).

[3] Dawson K G, Gomes D, Gerstein H, Blanchard J F, Kahler K H. The Economic Cost of Diabetes in Canada. Diab Care 1998;25:1303-7.

[4] Simpson SH, Corabian P, Jacobs P, et al. The cost of major comorbidity in people with diabetes mellitus. CMAJ 2003;168:1661-7.

[5] Goeree R, Morgan E. Lim, Rob Hopkins, et al. Prevalence, Total and Excess Costs of Diabetes and Related Complications in Ontario, Canada. CJD 2009;33(1):35-45.

[6] Lipscombe L, Hux J. Trends in diabetes prevalence, incidence and mortality in Ontario, Canada 1995-2005: a population-based study, Lancet 2007;369(9563):750-6.

[7] Wild S, Roglic G, Green A, Sicree R, King H. Global prevalence of diabetes: estimates for the year 2000 and projections for 2030. Diab Care 2004;27:1047-53.

[8] Centre for Disease Control and Prevention. Prevalence of Diabetes and Impaired fasting glucose in Adults – United States, 1999-2000 MMWR 2003;52.

[9] Hogan P, Dall T, Nikolov P; American Diabetes Association. Economic costs of diabetes in the US in 2002. Diab Care 2003;26(3):917-32.

[10] Leiter LA, Barr A, Belanger A, et al. Diabetes Screening in Canada (DIASCAN) Study: prevalence of undiagnosed diabetes and glucose intolerance in family physician offices. Diab Care 2001;24(6):1038-43.

[11] Fuller JH, Shipley MJ, Rose G, Jarrett RJ, Keen H. Coronary-heart-disease risk and impaired glucose tolerance. The Whitehall study. Lancet 1988;1:1373-6.

[12] Jarrett RJ, McCartney P, Keen H. The Bedford Survey: 10 year mortality rates in newly diagnosed diabetics, borderline diabetics and normoglycaemic controls and risk indices for coronary heart disease in borderline diabetics: Diabetologica 1982;22:79-84.

[13] Robins SJ, et al. The VA-HIT study Group. Relation of gemfibrozil treatment and lipid levels with major coronary events: VA-HIT: a randomized control trial. JAMA 2001 March;285(12):1585-91.

[14] Pan XR, Li GW, Hu YH, et al. Effects of diet and exercise in preventing NIDDM in people with impaired glucose tolerance. The Da Qing IGT and Diabetes Study. Diab Care 1997;20:537-44.

[15] Tuomilehto J, Lindstrom J, Eriksson JG, et al. Finnish Diabetes Prevention Study group. Prevention of type 2 diabetes mellitus by changes in lifestyle among subjects with impaired glucose tolerance. N Engl J Med 2001;344:1343-50.

[16] Knowler WC, Barrett-Conner E, Fowler SE, et al. Diabetes Prevention Program Research Group. Reduction in the incidence of type 2 diabetes with lifestyle intervention or metformin. N Engl J Med 2002;346;393-403.

[17] Larson H, Lindgarde F, Berglund G, Ahren B. Prediction of diabetes using ADA or WHO criteria in post-menopausal women: a 10-year follow- up study. Diabetologia 2004;43:1224-8.

[18] 2006 Census: Portrait of the Canadian Population in 2006, by Age and Sex: National portrait. Statistics Canada. Accessed November 8th 2010: http://www12.statcan.ca/census-recensement/2006/as-sa/97-551/p4-eng.cfm

[19] International Textbook of Diabetes Mellitus, 3rd Edition/2 Volume Set

[20] De Fronzo (Editor), Ele Ferrannini (Editor), Harry Keen (Editor), Paul Zimmet (Editor) Published by Wiley.

[21] Gillies C, Abrams K, Lambert P, et al. Pharmacological and lifestyle interventions to prevent or delay type 2 diabetes in people with impaired glucose tolerance: systematic review and meta-analysis. BMJ 2007;334:299.

[22] PHAC. PHAC Prediabetes and Diabetes Awareness in Canada (PADAC) Survey. 2009.

[23] WHO. Definition and diagnosis of diabetes mellitus and intermediate hyperglycemia. World Health Organization. 2006:1-50.

[24] Consequences of the new diagnostic criteria for DM in older men and women. The DECODE Study group. Diabetes Care 1999;22(10):1667-71.

[25] Gerstein H. Fasting versus Postload Glucose levels. Why the controversy? Diab Care 2001;24(11):1855-7.

[26] The DECODE-study group. Is fasting glucose sufficient to define diabetes? Epidemiological data from 20 European studies. European Diabetes Epidemiology Group. Diabetologica 2000;43(1):132-3.

[27] Tominaga M, Eguchi H, Manaka H, Igarashi K, Kato T, Sekikawa A. Impaired glucose tolerance is a risk factor for cardiovascular disease but not impaired fasting glucose: the Funagata Diabetes Study. Diab Care 1999;22(6):920-4.

[28] American Diabetes Association. Executive summary: standards of medical care in diabetes—2010. Diabetes Care 33: S4-S10.

[29] Goldenberg RM, Cheng AYY, Punthakee Z, Clement M. Position statement: Use of glycated hemoglobin (A1C) in the diagnosis of type 2 diabetes mellitus in adults. Can J Diabetes. 2011;35:247–249

[30] Wilson SE, Lipscombe LL, Rosella LC, Manuel DG: Trends in laboratory testing for diabetes in Ontario, Canada 1995-2005: A population-based study. BMC Hlth Serv Res 2009;9:41-47.

[31] Wilson SE, Rosella LC, Lipscombe LL, Manuel DG. The effectiveness and efficiency of diabetes screening in Ontario, Canada: a population-based cohort study. BMC Public Health 2010;10:506.

[32] Canadian Diabetes association [CDA] 2003 Clinical Practice Guidelines for the Prevention and Management of Diabetes in Canada. Cdn J Diabetes 2003;27:(s2).

[33] Canadian Diabetes Association Clinical Practice Guidelines Expert Committee. Canadian Diabetes Association 2008. Clinical practice guidelines for the prevention and management of diabetes in Canada. Can J Diabetes. 2008;32(suppl 1):S1-S201.

[34] Harris MI, Klein R, Welborn TA, Knuiman MW. Onset of NIDDM occurs at least 4-7 yr before clinical diagnosis. Diab Care 1992;15(7):815-9.

[35] Chiasson JL, Josse RG, Gomis R, Hanefeld M, Karasik A, Laakso M. Acarbose for prevention of type 2 diabetes mellitus: the STOP-NIDDM randomised trial. Lancet. 2002;359(9323):2072-7.

[36] Borch-Johnsen, Lauritzen T, Glumer C, Sandbaek A. Screening for Type 2 diabetes—should it be now? Diabet Med 2003;20:175–81.

[37] Ealovega MW, Tabaei BP, Brandle M, Burke R, Herman WH. Opportunistic screening for diabetes in routine clinical practice. Diab Care 2004;27(1):9-12.

[38] Alberti KG. Screening and diagnosis of prediabetes: where are we headed? Diabetes Obes Metab 2007;9 Suppl 1:12-6.

[39] Lindstrom J, Tuomilehto J. The Diabetes Risk Score. A practical tool to predict type 2 diabetes risk. Diab Care 2003;26:725-31.

[40] Kaczorowoski J, Robinson C, Nerenberg K. Development of the CANRISK quesiton-naire to screen for prediabetes and undiagnosed type 2 diabetes. Cdn J Diabetes 2009;33(4):318-85.

[41] Nerenberg K, Punthakee Z, Gerstein H. Systematic review of screening quesiton-naires for type 2 diabetes. Clinical Investigative Medicine. 2006;(29):314.

[42] Harris R, et al. Screening Adults for type 2 diabetes: a review of the evidence for the US preventive services task force. Annals of Int Med 2003;138(3);4.

[43] Tabaei BP, et al. Community based screening for diabetes in Michigan. Diab Care 2003;26(3):668-70.

[44] Lawrence JM, Bennet P, Young A, Robinson AM. Screening for diabetes in general practice: cross sectional population study. BMJ 2001;323(7312):548-51.

[45] Tsuyuki RT, Johnson JA, Teo KK, et al. A Randomized Trial of the Effect of Com-munity Pharmacist Intervention on Cholesterol Risk Management: The Study of Car-diovascular Risk Intervention by Pharmacists (SCRIP). Arch Intern Med 2002;162:1149-55.

[46] Grant T, et al. Community based screening for cardiovascular disease and diabetes using HbA1c. Am J Prev Med 2004;26(4):271-5.

[47] Feig D, Palda VA, Lipscombe L with The Canadian Task Force on Preventive Health Care. Screening for type 2 diabetes mellitus to prevent vascular complications. CMAJ 2005;172(2):177-80.

[48] Gulli C, Lunau K. Adding Fuel to the Doctor Crisis: Five million Canadians are cur-rently without a family doctor – and things are only getting worse.. Maclean's [Busi-ness Magazine], 14 January 2008, p. 62.

[49] Agarwal G. How to diagnose diabetes. CMAJ. 2005;172(5):615-6.

[50] Ciardulli LM, Goode JV. Using health observances to promote wellness in communi-ty pharmacies. J Am Pharm Assoc (Wash). 2003 Jan-Feb;43(1):13-6.

[51] Park P, Sargeant L, Griffin S, Wareham N. The performance of a risk score in detect-ing undiagnosed hyperglycemia. Diab Care June 2002;25(6):984-88.

[52] Agarwal G, Kaczorowski, J, Gerstein, H, Hanna S. Effectiveness of a community-based diabetes program to increase awareness and detection of diabetes. North American Primary Care Research Group (NAPCRG), Montreal, Quebec, Canada. No-vember 2009. [Abstract]

[53] Waugh N, Scotland G, McNamee P, et al. Screening for type 2 diabetes: literature re-view and economic modelling. Health Technol Assess 2007;11(17):iii-iv, ix-xi, 1-125.

[54] Health Technology Assessment. HTA Reports and Publications. Health Technology Update. Issue 12; November 2009. Accessed Sept 28th 2010; http://www.cadth.ca/index.php/en/hta/reports-publications/health-technology-update/ht-update-12/diabetes-screening-and-diagnosis.

[55] Rosella LC, Manuel D, Burchill C, Stukel TA. A population-based risk algorithm for the development of diabetes: development and validation of the Diabetes Population Risk Tool (DPoRT). J Epidemiol Community Health 2011;65(7):613-20.

Chapter 2

Lifestyle Modification Is the First Line Treatment for Type 2 Diabetes

Kazuko Masuo

Additional information is available at the end of the chapter

1. Introduction

The prevalence of diabetes, especially type 2 diabetes and hypertension are significantly increased with the prevalence of obesity (Figures 1, 2 and 3) [1, 2]. Type 2 diabetes, hypertension frequently associated with type 2 diabetes, and obesity are important risk factors for cardiovascular morbidity and mortality and cardiac- and renal complications. Hyperglycemia as well as hyperinsulinemia in type 2 diabetes is a cardiovascular risk by itself [3]. Type 2 diabetes, hypertension and obesity are characterized by stimulation of the renin-angiotensin-aldosterone system (RAAS), elevated sympathetic activity and insulin resistance. Importantly, these characteristics, themselves, are one of the cardiovascular risks. Therefore, pharmacological and non-pharmacological treatments for type 2 diabetes should be selected from favourable effects on stimulated RAAS, elevated sympathetic nervous system activity, insulin resistance and leptin resistance.

Weight loss is recommended to delay and prevent type 2 diabetes in obesity, and for the treatment. Lifestyle modification such as a caloric restricted diet, reducing sedentary behaviour and an increase in exercise form the basis of all therapy. Weight loss treated with lifestyle modification including calorie restriction and/or exercise causes normalization of stimulated RAAS, sympathetic activation, insulin resistance, and hyperleptinemia, which are usually observed in type 2 diabetes and obesity. Recently, Straznicky et al. [4] and Masuo et al. [5] have shown the low caloric diet and exercise have different effects on insulin resistance, the RAAS, and sympathetic nervous activity in obese hypertensive subjects, although similar weight loss was observed between both interventions. Straznicky et al. [4] reported that exercise had stronger effects of normalized the RAAS stimulation, sympathetic activation and insulin resistance compared to diet only, whereas Masuo et al. [5] showed mild calorie restriction and mild exercise has different mechanisms on weight loss (normalization on sympathetic

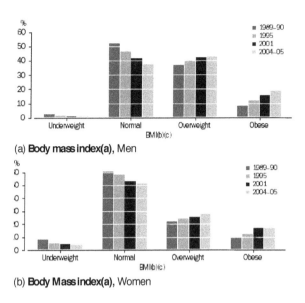

(a) **Body mass index(a)**, Men

(b) **Body Mass index(a)**, Women

Source: National Health Survey, Australian Bureau of Statics in 2008.
Prevalence of overweight and obesity has increased in both genders.

Figure 1. Overweight/obesity has increased in both genders in Australia [Source. Australian Bureau of Statics. 4819.0. Released at 11:30 AM (CANBERRA TIME) 25/01/2008] Reference [1]

activation for mild calorie restriction, and normalization on insulin resistance for exercise). The observations, however, demonstrate that a combination therapy for weight loss with a low caloric diet and exercise is recommended for weight loss due to stronger suppression of insulin resistance and sympathetic activation, which both are known as strong risk factors for cardiovascular events. Although few studies have observed changes in body weight, blood pressure, neurohormonal changes over a long duration such as 2 years, Masuo *et al.* [6] observed more than 30% individuals who initially succeeded to significantly lose weight, had rebound weight gain over 2 years. Understanding mechanisms underlying both type 2 diabetes and obesity may help to achieve weight loss and maintenance of weight loss and the stricter blood glucose goal. Maintenance of weight loss is another key factor to reduce cardiovascular risks in type 2 diabetes in obesity [6].

In addition, most hypertensive patients with diabetes and obesity are very resistant to controlling hypertension and frequently require two or more types of medications to achieve blood pressure goals. Similarly, diabetic patients, especially type 2 diabetic patients with obesity, need higher dose of anti-diabetic medications such as metformin or insulin. However, pharmacological treatments for hypertension and diabetes with weight loss could reduce pharmacological treatment [7, 8].

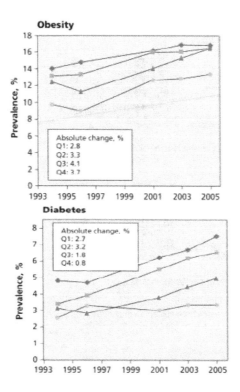

Figure 2. Prevalence of diabetes has increased in parallel with obesity. [Reference 2]

The purpose of this review is to provide, *i*) the importance of lifestyle modifications to delay and prevent type 2 diabetes, *ii*) Lifestyle modification to reduce cardiovascular risks in type 2 diabetes, and *iii*) weight loss for the better pharmacological control on type 2 diabetes and hypertension, which frequently co-exist with type 2 diabetes. *iv*) The mode of weight loss influences different physiological pathways, with calorie restriction and exercise program. *v*) Different mechanisms may contribute to reductions in blood pressure and cardiovascular risks associated with weight loss with the relevant physiological mechanisms at play being dependent on the mode of weight loss.

2. Type 2 diabetes versus Type 1 diabetes

Prevalence of diabetes has increased markedly over the last 20 years in parallel with obesity (Figures 2 and 3) [1, 2]. As of 2010 there are approximately 285 million people with the disease compared to around 30 million in 1985. Long-term complications from high blood sugar can include heart disease, strokes, renal failure, diabetic retinopathy, and diabetic neuropathy.

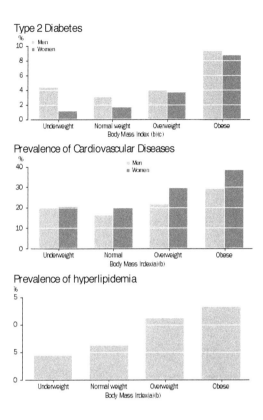

Figure 3. Prevalence of type 2 diabetes, cardiovascular disease and hyperlipidemia (hyper cholesterolemia) increased with obesity in both genders. [Source: National Health Survey, Australia, 2004-2005] Reference [1]

Diabetes mellitus includes type 2 diabetes (formerly noninsulin dependent diabetes), type 1 diabetes (formerly insulin dependent diabetes), and gestational diabetes. These 3 types of diabetes have different characteristics and progress [9]. Ninety percent of diabetic patients are type 2 diabetes and the other 10% are due primarily to diabetes mellitus type 1 and gestational diabetes.

2.1. Diabetes mellitus type 2 (Formerly noninsulin-dependent diabetes mellitus (NIDDM))

Type 2 diabetes is the most common form of diabetes, affecting 90% of all patients with diabetes. This type of diabetes is characterised by metabolic disorder with insulin resistance and relative insulin deficiency [10]. This is in contrast to type 1 diabetes, in which there is an absolute insulin deficiency due to destruction of islet cells in the pancreas [9, 11]. Obesity is thought to be the primary cause of type 2 diabetes in people who are genetically predisposed to the disease, and obesity has been found to contribute to approximately 55% of case of type 2 diabetes [12].

The disease is strongly genetic in origin but lifestyle factors such as excess weight, inactivity, high blood pressure and poor diet are major risk factors for its development. Symptoms may not show for many years and, by the time they appear, significant problems may have developed. People with type 2 diabetes are twice as likely to suffer cardiovascular disease. The classic symptoms are excess thirst, frequent urination, and constant hunger.

Type 2 diabetes is initially managed by increasing exercise and dietary modification. If blood glucose levels are not adequately lowered by these measures, medications such as metformin or insulin may be needed. In those on insulin, there is typically the requirement to routinely check blood sugar levels.

2.2. Type 1 diabetes (Insulin-dependent diabetes)

Type 1 diabetes is an auto-immune disease targeting on the insulin-producing beta cells in the pancreas. This type of diabetes, also known as juvenile-onset diabetes, accounts for approximately 10% of all people with the disease. In the majority of cases this type of diabetes appears before the patient is 40 years old, triggered by environmental factors such as viruses, diet or chemicals in people genetically predisposed. Patients with type 1 diabetes will require insulin therapy regularly, and should follow a careful diet and exercise plan.

2.3. Gestational diabetes mellitus

Gestational diabetes, or glucose intolerance, is first diagnosed during pregnancy through an oral glucose tolerance test. Between 5.5 and 8.8% of pregnant women develop gestational diabetes in Australia [13], and 2 to 10 percent of all pregnancies in USA [14]. The hormones produced during pregnancy increase the amount of insulin needed to control blood glucose levels. If the body can't meet this increased need for insulin, women can develop gestational diabetes during the late stages of pregnancy.

While the glucose intolerance usually returns to normal after the birth, the mother has a significant risk of developing permanent diabetes while the baby is more likely to develop obesity and impaired glucose tolerance and/or diabetes later in life [15]. Risk factors for gestational diabetes include a family history of diabetes, increasing maternal age, obesity, lack of sleep [16], and being a member of a community or ethnic group with a high risk of developing type 2 diabetes. Self-care and dietary changes are essential in treatment.

3. Prevalence of type 2 diabetes

The prevalence of type 2 diabetes has dramatically increased in parallel in rising prevalence of obesity (Figures 1 and 2), and it increases with obesity (Figure 3). Rates of diabetes in 1985 in worldwide were estimated at 30 million, increasing to 135 million in 1995 and 217 million

	Type 1 Diabetes	Type 2 Diabetes
Diagnosis:	Genetic, environmental and auto-immune factors, idiopathic	Genetic, obesity (central adipose), physical inactivity, high/low birth weight, GDM, poor placental growth, metabolic syndrome
Warning Signs:	Increased thirst & urination, constant hunger, weight loss, blurred vision and extreme tiredness, glycouria	Feeling tired or ill, frequent urination (especially at night), unusual thirst, weight loss, blurred vision, frequent infections and slow wound healing, asymptomatic
Target Groups:	Children/teens	Adults, elderly, ethnic groups
Prone ethnic groups:	All	more common in African American, Latino/Hispanic, indigenous, Asian or Pacific Islander
Bodily Effects:	Believed to be triggered autoimmune destruction of the beta cells; autoimmune attack may occur following a viral infection such as mumps, rubella cytomegalovirus	Appears to be related to aging, sedentary life-style, genetic influence, but mostly obesity
Common physical attributes found:	Mostly Normal or Thin	Mostly Overweight or Obese
You have this when:	Your body makes too little or no insulin.	Your body either cannot produce insulin or does not use it properly.
Estimated percentage of occurrence:	5% -10% of the 171 million of people affected by diabetes in 2000	90% - 95%-of total cases. Although the projected number of Americans that will have type II diabetes in the year 2030 will double from 171 million to 366 million cases
Affected age group:	Between 5 - 25 (maximum numbers in this age group; Type 1 can affect at any age)	Until recently, the only type of diabetes that was common in children was Type 1 diabetes, most children who have Type 2 diabetes have a family history of diabetes, are overweight, and are not very physically active. Usually develops around puberty
Glucose Channels/receptors:	Open and absorb glucose into cell to be utilized by processes after the induction of insulin	Are unable to open and absorb glucose, therefore glucose cannot be utilized by processes; as a result the glucose stays in the blood stream
Cure:	None	Physical exercise, healthy loss of weight & diet control
Treatment:	Insulin Injections, dietary plan, regular check up of blood sugar levels, daily exercise Goals: optimal glucose, prevent/treat chronic complications, enhance health with food/PA, individual nutrition needs	Diet, exercise, weight loss, and in many cases medication. Insulin Injections may also be used, SMBG
Dependency:	Insulin-dependent	Not insulin-dependent
Onset:	Rapid (weeks)	Slow (years)

[Reference, American Diabetes Association-Executive Summary-2012, A-348]

Table 1. Comparison between type 1 diabetes and type 2 diabetes

in 2005 [17]. This increase is believed to be primarily due to the global population aging, a decrease in exercise, and increasing rates of obesity [18].

The prevalence of diabetes is recognized as a global epidemic by the World Health Organization (WHO) [19]. The World Health Organization (WHO) has reported 346 million people worldwide had diabetes in 2004. Globally as of 2010 it was estimated that there were 285 million people with type 2 diabetes, and this is equivalent to about 6% of the world's adult population [18]. In 2010, diabetic patients were estimated as 316 million people worldwide, and this is equivalent to about 6% of the world's adult population. Importantly, the National Diabetes Fact Sheet 2011 by Centers for Disease Control and Prevention (CDC) pointed out 7.0 million American people (27% of those with diabetes) were not diagnosed and an estimated 79 million Americans have pre-diabetes, indication that much more of the population were affected by diabetes [20, 21]. An estimated 3.4 million people died from consequences of diabetes in 2004, which more than 80% of diabetes deaths occurs in low- and middle-income countries, and diabetes deaths will increase by double between 2005 and 2030 [22]. The five countries with the greatest number of people with diabetes as of 2000 are India, China, the United States, Indonesia, and Japan. Diabetes is common both in the developed and the developing world, but not in the underdeveloped world. Women seem to be at a greater risk as do certain ethnic groups such as South Asians, Pacific Islanders, Latinos, and Native Americans [18]. This may be due to enhanced sensitivity to a Western lifestyle in certain ethnic groups [23].

4. What causes type 2 diabetes?

Many epidemiological studies showed a strong association between obesity and type 2 diabetes, however it is also true that not all obese individuals have type 2 diabetes [20]. Majority of the onset and development of type 2 diabetes is caused by a combination of lifestyle and genetics. Other confounders are also reported to relate to the onset and development of type 2 diabetes: i.e. lack of sleep [16], which has been linked to type 2 diabetes through its effect on metabolism [15], nutritional status of a mother during fetal development may also play a role, with one proposed mechanism being that of altered DNA methylation [24]. While some are under personal control, such as diet and obesity, others, such as increasing age, female gender, and genetic susceptibility, is not. The followings are several causes known for type 2 diabetes.

4.1. Lifestyle

A number of lifestyle factors are known to be important to the development of type 2 diabetes, including obesity, lack of physical activity (sedentary life style) [12], poor diet, stress, and urbanization.

Excess body fat is associated with 30% of cases in type 2 diabetes of Chinese and Japanese descent, 60-80% of cases in those of European and African descent, and 100% of Pima Indians and Pacific Islanders [19, 23]. Interestingly, Pima Indians and Pacific Islanders have relatively higher waist-to-hip ratio even if they are not obese, suggesting that abdominal obesity and visceral fat is more important to cause type 2 diabetes.

Dietary factors also influence the risk of developing type 2 diabetes. Consumption of sugar-sweetened drinks in excess is associated with an increased risk. It has been demonstrated saturated fat and trans-fatty acids increase LDL cholesterol, the risk of type 2 diabetes, and cardiovascular risk. Poly-unsaturated, and monounsaturated fat decreasing the risk, but It is recommended to take both in a limited quantity. The American Heart Association has recommended that Americans should limit their intake of saturated fats to 7% of their total calories in a day, while unsaturated fats can form 30% of the calorie intake.

4.2. Genetics

Most cases of diabetes involve many genes, with each being a small contributor to an increased probability of becoming a type 2 diabetic. If one identical twin has diabetes, the chance of the other developing diabetes within his lifetime is greater than 90% while the rate for non-identical siblings is 25-50%. As of 2011, more than 36 genes have been found that contribute to the risk of type 2 diabetes. All of these genes together still only account for 10% of the total heritable component of the disease. The TCF7L2 allele, for example, increases the risk of developing diabetes by 1.5 times and is the greatest risk of the common genetic variants. Most of the genes linked to diabetes are involved in beta cell functions in pancreas.

There are a number of rare cases of diabetes that arise due to an abnormality in a single gene (known as monogenic forms of diabetes or "other specific types of diabetes"). These include maturity onset diabetes of the young (MODY), Donohue syndrome, and Rabson-Mendenhall syndrome, among others. Maturity onset diabetes of the young constitutes 1–5% of all cases of diabetes in young people.

4.3. Medical conditions

There are a number of medications, including glucocorticoids, thiazides, beta blockers, atypical antipsychotics, and statins that can predispose to diabetes [25].

Statins have beneficial effects on reductions of cardiovascular risks through lipids control, and mortality and morbidity in patients with high cardiac risk such as diabetes, coronary heart disease, ischemic heart disease, chronic kidney disease, chronic heart failure, and peripheral vascular disease [26, 27]. National and international clinical guidelines in the management of these cardiovascular disease conditions all advocate for the utilization of statins therapy in appropriate patients. The meta-analysis including 80,771 participants with low cardiac risk showed that all-cause mortality was significantly lower among patients receiving a statin than among controls with a 10-year risk of cardiovascular disease < 20% [28]. Patients in the statin group were also significantly less likely than controls to have nonfatal myocardial infarction, and nonfatal stroke, but the effects did not depend on high- and low-potency statins, or larger reductions in cholesterol. The JUPITER trial [27] and Atherosclerosis Risk in Communities (ARIC) Study [29] demonstrated that suppression of low-grade inflammation by statins improves these clinical outcomes.

Recently, concerns were raised regarding the onset and development of diabetes in statin-treated patients [30]. The meta-analysis studied by Coleman *et al.* [31] showed that statins, as a class, did not demonstrate a statistically significant positive or negative impact on a patient's risk of developing new-onset type 2 diabetes mellitus, whereas Satter et al. [32] observed that statin therapy is associated with a slightly increased risk of development of diabetes using meta-analysis, but the risk is low both in absolute terms and when compared with the reduction in coronary events. Clinical practice in patients with moderate or high cardiovascular risk or existing cardiovascular disease should not change. In 2012, two major studies have addressed the question of whether statins lead to an increase in diabetes, which included the meta-analysis of 33,000 participants enrolled in 5 major clinical trials using statins [33, 34], and analysed data from 153,840 postmenopausal women between 50 and 80 years in the Women Health Initiative Study [30]. The study showed women taking statins had a 48% increased risk of diabetes compared those without statins. The American Heart Association concluded in 2012 that the benefits of statins on lipids-lowering effects and resultant reductions in cardiovascular risks overweighted to the new onset or development of diabetes [35].

Combined bezafibrate/statin therapy is theoretically believed more effective in achieving a comprehensive lipid control and residual cardiovascular risk reduction [36, 37]. The ACCORD Study [38], however, showed that the combination of fenofibrate and simvastatin did not reduce the rate of fatal cardiovascular events, nonfatal myocardial infarction, or nonfatal stroke, as compared with simvastatin alone. Based on the beneficial effects of pan-PPAR agonist bezafibrate on glucose metabolism and prevention of new-onset diabetes, one could expect a neutralization of the adverse pro-diabetic effect of statins using the strategy of a combined statin/fibrate therapy [39, 40].

5. Type 2 diabetes mellitus as a risk factor for cardiovascular disease

Several epidemiological studies are available to understand that diabetes is a strong cardiovascular disease risks. A population-based European Prospective Investigation into Cancer and Nutrition (EPIC)-Potsdam study [41], which consisted of 23,455 participants (9,729 men and 15,438 women) followed up from 1994-1998 to 2006, showed that participants with a high risk of the development of diabetes had significantly higher risks of myocardial infarction and stroke than those with a low risk of diabetes development. Subjects at a high risk of diabetes development were also at considerably higher risks of developing cardiovascular complications in general.

The Framingham Heart Study [42] observed that both cardiovascular disease and non-cardiovascular disease mortality rates among individuals with diabetes mellitus were approximately 2-fold higher compared with individuals without diabetes. Non-cardiovascular disease mortality declined among women without diabetes mellitus, while no change in non-cardiovascular disease mortality was observed among women and men with diabetes between the "1950 to 1975" and "1976 to 2001" period. Importantly, individuals with diabetes were at a higher risk of all-cause mortality, especially cardiovascular disease mortality, in both the periods compared to those without diabetes. Another study has shown that diabetes is associated with a substantial increase in all cause and coronary heart disease mortality [43].

Regarding the gender differences in mortality and morbidity of cardiovascular complications, Kanaya *et al.* [44], in their meta-analysis, documented that absolute coronary heart disease death rates were higher in diabetic men compared with diabetic women at every age except the very oldest, however, the excess relative risk of coronary heart disease mortality in women versus men with diabetes was absent after adjusting for classic coronary heart disease risk factors (*i.e.* dyslipidemia, hypertension).

Recently, the Detection of Ischemia in Asymptomatic Diabetics (DIAD) study [45] was performed in 1,123 patients with type 2 diabetes and no symptoms of coronary heart disease using adenosine-stress radionuclide myocardial perfusion imaging from 2000 to 2007. The cumulative cardiac event rate in DIAD was 2.9% over a mean follow-up of 4.8 years for an average of 0.6% per year, which is higher compared to the general population.

The World Health Organization Multinational Study of Vascular Disease in diabetes [46, 47] examined the relationship between excess mortality and proteinuria/hypertension in a stratified random sample of 4,714 diabetic patients aged 35-55 years from 1975 to 1987. Even in the absence of proteinuria and hypertension, standardized mortality rates were significant higher in patients with both type 1 and type 2 diabetes compared to the general population. Standardized mortality was higher in those with type 1 diabetes compared with type 2 diabetes, and the standard mortality rate increased with increasing diabetes duration. In addition, both hypertension and proteinuria had a strikingly high mortality risk by 11-fold for men with type 1 diabetes, and 5 fold for men with type 2 diabetes, indicating that diabetes accompanying cardiovascular disease leads to even higher mortality risk.

Hypertension is twice as frequent in diabetic patients in the general population, and its prevalence is higher in type 2 diabetes than in type 1 diabetes. In type 2 diabetes, the onset of hypertension often precedes the diagnosis of diabetes, whereas in type 1 diabetes it is strictly related to the presence of nephropathy [48].

Further, many studies have shown the strong associations of myocardial infarction [49] and atherosclerosis [50-52]. A number of epidemiological studies provide evidence that diabetes mellitus is a significant risk factor for cardiovascular disease mortality and morbidity [53]. Longer duration of diabetes is a stronger predictor of mortality among diabetic patients. Therefore, people who have diabetes mellitus or strong lifestyle or dietary factors to predict the development of type 2 diabetes [54] should avoid the cardiovascular complications.

6. Neurohoromonal characteristics in type 2 diabetes: Insulin resistance and sympathetic activity

It is widely recognized that insulin resistance is a major mechanism of the onset of type 2 diabetes. Insulin resistance in children could predict future glucose intolerance and type 2 diabetes in 10 years [46, 55]. Reduced energy expenditure and resting metabolic rate are predictive of weight gain (obesity). The sympathetic nervous system participates in regulating energy balance through thermogenesis. Many epidemiological and clinical studies have shown a close relationship between sympathetic nervous system activity and insulin levels in obesity and in weight gain [56, 57]. Elevations of sympathetic nervous system activity and insulin levels during weight gain [58-60] and reductions of sympathetic activity and insulin levels during weight loss [61-64] are typically observed. In addition, The response of the sympathetic nervous system to changes in plasma insulin levels after oral glucose loading (oral glucose tolerance test) are different between subjects with and without insulin resistance [65], between nonobese and obese subjects [66], and between subjects with and without metabolic syndrome [67]. Those observations provide evidence of a strong linkage between the activity of the sympathetic nervous system and insulin levels over glucose metabolisms. Straznicky *et al.* [68] reported that the progress from metabolic syndrome to type 2 diabetes might be associated with increased central sympathetic drive, blunted sympathetic responsiveness, and altered norepinephrine disposition.

Acute hyperglycemia caused sympathetic activation and peripheral vasodilation. Moreover, both acute and chronic hyperglycemia and hyperinsulinemia may enhance adrenergic vasoconstriction and decrease vasodilation in animal models (pithed rats) [69, 70]. Insulin causes forearm vasoconstriction in obese, insulin-resistant hypertensive humans [71]. On the other hand, van Veen *et al.* [72] found that hyperglycemia in the forearm induced vasodilation, but this vasodilation was not modified by hyperinsulinemia.

Huggett *et al.* [66] examined muscle sympathetic nerve activity (MSNA) in four groups of subjects, patients with essential hypertension and type 2 diabetes, patients with type 2 diabetes alone, patients with essential hypertension alone, and healthy normotensive controls. They found higher MSNA in hypertensive-type 2 diabetic patients compared with hypertensive alone patients or type 2 diabetic alone patients, and higher MSNA in hypertensive alone patients or type 2 diabetic alone patients compared with healthy normotensive controls. Fasting insulin levels were greater in hypertensive-type 2 diabetic patients and type 2 diabetic patients compared to hypertensive patients or healthy normotensive subjects. These findings provided evidence that type 2 diabetic patients had elevated sympathetic nerve activity regardless of the prevailing blood pressure levels, and that the combination of hypertension and type 2 diabetes resulted in an augmentation in sympathetic nerve activity and levels of plasma insulin.

Moreover, stimulation of the renin-angiotensin-aldosterone system (RAAS) is frequently demonstrated in type 2 diabetes [73], and may be related to insulin resistance either via direct or indirect mechanisms [74].

7. Treatments for type 2 diabetes

Weight loss is recommended as the first line of treatment for type 2 diabetes and hypertension associated with obesity, because obesity is the primary cause for insulin resistance, metabolic syndrome and type 2 diabetes. Indeed, lifestyle modification including a low caloric diet, reducing sedentary behaviour and exercise form the foundation of all therapy. For the subjects who are more severely obese or unable to undertake an exercise program, bariatric surgery is recommended.

7.1. Lifestyle modification for weight loss

Weight loss is recommended as the first-line treatment for obesity-related type 2 diabetes and hypertension. The objective of treatment for obesity, type 2 diabetes and hypertension is both to reduce the high risk of cardiovascular events and to prevent or delay the onset of type 2 diabetes and complications. Lifestyle intervention with diet and exercise leading to weight loss prevents and delays the onset of type 2 diabetes or glucose intolerance [75]. Weight loss may also prevent cardiovascular- and renal-complications [76-79], and renal function and left ventricular hypertrophy as a marker for future cardiac events in obese individuals with metabolic syndrome and hypertension [77, 80]. The US Diabetes Prevention Program [81] and the Oslo Diet and Exercise Study [82] have shown marked clinical benefits with lifestyle intervention, and modest weight loss, on the resolution of the metabolic syndrome and type 2 diabetes. A limited number of epidemiological studies have shown that intentional weight loss may be associated with increased mortality and fat loss may reduce the all-cause mortality rate [83].

Cohort studies with lifestyle intervention [84] and case control studies with bariatric surgeries [85, 86] also provide some evidence that intentional weight loss has long-term benefits on all cause mortality in overweight adults. In a cohort of patients enrolled in a cardiac rehabilitation program, weight loss was associated with favourable long-term outcomes on the composite end-point of mortality and acute cardiovascular events (fatal and nonfatal myocardial infarction, fatal and nonfatal stroke, emergent revascularization for unstable angina pectoris, and congestive heart failure) [87].

Many clinical studies have demonstrated that weight loss associated with life-style modification adds to the first line treatment for diabetes mellitus and the efficacy of antihypertensive pharmacological treatments [8], however, maintaining weight loss is often the greatest challenge [5, 6, 88].

7.1.1. Calorie restricted diet versus aerobic exercise

The American Diabetes Association (ADA) has recommended for the maintenance of a healthy weight to prevent and control diabetes as following; (i) more than 2.5 hours of exercise per week, (ii) having a modest fat intake (approximately 30% of energy supply), and (iii) rating sufficient fiber [89]. Recently, several investigations [4, 5, 90] compared the effects on weight loss between calorie restriction (diet) and exercise. They showed that combined intervention with diet and exercise proved to be effective in weight reduction than diet alone or exercise alone. Masuo et al. [5] reported that the group with mild exercise alone had greater and faster loss of total body fat-mass compared to the diet alone group, whereas Toji et al. [90] reported that exercise intervention alone was not found to be effective on weight loss. There are discordant results on the effects of diet and exercise on weight loss and weight loss-induced blood pressure reductions, however many large cohort interventions and clinical studies have

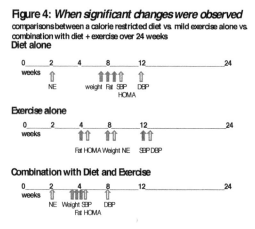

Figure 4: *When significant changes were observed*
comparisons between a calorie restricted diet vs. mild exercise alone vs.
combination with diet + exercise over 24 weeks
Diet alone

Exercise alone

Combination with Diet and Exercise

Reference [5]
NE, plasma norepinephrine as index of sympathetic activity;
HOMA, HOMA-IR (homeostasis model assessment of insulin resistance) as an index of insulin resistance; Weight, body weight; Fat, total body fat-mass; SBP, systolic blood pressure;
DBP, diastolic blood pressure.

Figure 4. When significant chages were observed comparisons between a calorie restricted diet vs. mild exercise alone vs. combination with diet + exercise over 24 weeks

shown combination weight loss regimens with mild calorie restriction and mild exercise was the most effective for significant weight loss compared to diet alone or exercise alone.

A low caloric diet and exercise exert different effects on insulin resistance, the RAAS, and sympathetic nervous activity in obese hypertensive subjects, even though similar weight loss was observed [4, 5]. Low caloric diet may be prominent for normalization of sympathetic nervous activity and exercise may be related more to normalization of insulin resistance [5, 88] (Figure 4). They previously observed that baseline plasma norepinephrine levels could predict future weight gain and weight gain-induced blood pressure elevation over 5 years in a longitudinal study [91], resistant weight loss by weight loss intervention with combination of calorie restriction and exercise intervention over 2 years. [6, 88] Similarly, Straznicky *et al.* [92] showed baseline sympathetic tone measured by muscle sympathetic nervous activity and nutritional responsiveness could predict the success of dietary weight loss, but not exercise, supporting the results including that the sympathetic nervous activity plays major mechanisms and roles on diet-induced weight loss pointed by Masuo, *et al.* [5]. Ribeiro *et al.* [93], Trombetta *et al.* [94] and Tonacio *et al.* [95] compared the effects of a low caloric diet and exercise on blood pressure lowering and forearm blood flow. They observed that only exercise, not diet, significantly increased forearm blood flow.

Santarpia *et al.* [96] reviewed the effectiveness of weight loss regimens and body composition after weight loss between diet and exercise. At a long term follow up (over one year), relatively high protein, moderately low calorie, low glycemic index diets, associated with a daily, moderate intensity, physical exercise (of at least 30 min), appear to be more successful in limiting long term rebound, maintaining fat-free-mass and achieving the highest fat loss. Diet alone or physical exercise alone does not produce similar results. Adequate dietetic advice plus regular physical exercise avoid the fat-free-mass loss usually observed in the rebound of the weight cycling syndrome and prevent the onset of sarcopenic obesity.

Exercise training is important for weight loss and to prevent rebound weight gain after significant weight loss. Public health interventions promoting walking are likely to be the most successful. Indeed, walking is unique because of its safety, accessibility, and popularity. It is noteworthy that there is a clear dissociation between the adaptation of cardiopulmonary fitness and the improvements in the metabolic risk profile such as insulin resistance and sympathetic activation, which can be induced by endurance training programs. Dumortier *et al.* [97] also reported that individualized low intensity endurance aerobic training improves lipid oxidation, body composition and insulin resistance. It appears that as long as the increase in energy expenditure is sufficient, low-intensity endurance exercise is likely to generate beneficial metabolic effects that would be essentially similar to those produced by high-intensity exercise [98]. The clinician should therefore focus on the improvement of the metabolic profile rather than on weight loss alone [98].

7.1.2. Dietary

7.1.2.1. Saturated fat versus unsaturated fat

Recently, several large cohort studies have shown that saturated fat, which comes mainly from animal sources of food, raises LDL cholesterol and links strongly to cardiovascular risk [99, 100]. Saturated fats are needed for the production of hormones, the stabilization of cellular membranes, the padding around organs, and for energy. A deficiency in the consumption of saturated fats can lead to age-related declines in white blood cell function, along with dysfunction of the immune system and cancer [101]; however, a high content of saturated fat can leads to coronary heart disease [102], ischemic heart disease, and atherosclerosis and increase the chances of stroke.

Consistent evidence from prospective observational studies of habitual trans fatty acids (TFA) consumption and retrospective observational studies using TFA biomarkers indicates that TFA consumption increases risk of clinical coronary heart disease, and other disease outcomes such as cancer [102].

Unsaturated fats are known to increase the levels of High Density Lipoprotein (HDL cholesterol) and hence decrease LDL and VLDL cholesterol. Both types of unsaturated fat- mono-unsaturated and poly-unsaturated fats can replace saturated fats in the diet. Substituting saturated fats with unsaturated fats help to lower levels of total cholesterol and LDL cholesterol in the blood. However, intake of unsaturated fats in very high amounts can also increase the risk of coronary heart diseases.

i.   **Monounsaturated fat:** This is a type of fat found in a variety of foods and oils. Studies show that eating foods rich in monounsaturated fats (MUFAs) improves blood cholesterol levels, which can decrease the risk of heart disease. Research also shows that MUFAs may benefit insulin levels and blood sugar control, which can be especially helpful for type 2 diabetes.

ii.　**Polyunsaturated fat (PUFAs):** This is a type of fat found mostly in plant-based foods and oils. The Swedish Mammography Cohort study including 34, 670 women with a mean follow-up of 10.4 years, showed that intake of long-chain omega-3 PUFAs is inversely associated with risk of stroke, whereas dietary cholesterol is positively associated with risk [103]. Similarly, Chowdhury *et al.* [104] observed in meta-analysis that moderate, inverse associations of fish consumption and long chain omega 3 fatty acids with cerebrovascular risk, but long chain omega 3 fatty acids measured as circulating biomarkers in observational studies or supplements in primary and secondary prevention trials were not associated with cerebrovascular disease. The beneficial effect of fish intake on cerebrovascular risk is likely to be mediated through the interplay of a wide range of nutrients abundant in fish. PUFAs decrease the risk of type 2 diabetes. One type of polyunsaturated fat, a long chain omega-3 fatty acids is especially beneficial to coronary heart disease.

iii.　**Trans-fatty acids (TFA):** Growing evidence indicates that trans-fatty acids (TFA) adversely affect cardiovascular health. Controlled trials and observational studies provide concordant evidence that consumption of TFA from partially hydrogenated oils adversely affects multiple cardiovascular risk factors, and contributes significantly to increased risk of coronary heart disease events. The public health implications of ruminant TFA consumption appear much more limited. Nurses' health study showed that *trans*-fat intake was associated with increased risk of coronary heart disease, particularly for younger women [105]. Interestingly, incidence of insulin resistance is lowered with diets higher in monounsaturated fats (especially oleic acid), while the opposite is true for diets high in polyunsaturated fats (especially large amounts of arachidonic acid) as well as saturated fats. This relationship between dietary fats and insulin resistance is presumed secondary to the relationship between insulin resistance and inflammation, which is partially modulated by dietary fat ratios (Omega3/6/9) with both omega 3 and 9 thought to be anti-inflammatory, and omega 6 pro-inflammatory [106].

It is recommended to take both in a limited quantity. The American Heart Association has recommended that Americans should limit their intake of saturated fats to 7% of their total calories in a day, while unsaturated fats can form 30% of the calorie intake to reduced cardiovascular risks.

7.1.2.2. Special diet

i.　**Low Carbohydrate Diet**

Low-carbohydrate diets are dietary programs that restrict carbohydrate consumption usually for weight control or for the treatment of obesity. The term "low-carbohydrate diet" is generally applied to diets that restrict carbohydrates to less than 20% of caloric intake, but can also refer to diets that simply restrict or limit carbohydrates. Recently, the low carbohydrate diets has been spotlighted due to strong effects on weight loss, but many investigations have also shown no benefits on the reductions on cardiovascular risk as the major aim of weight loss.

A study of more than 100,000 people over more than 20 years within "the Nurses' Health Study" observationally concluded that a low-carbohydrate diet high in vegetables, with a large proportion of proteins and oils coming from plant sources, decreases mortality with a hazard ratio of 0.8. In contrast, a low-carbohydrate diet with largely animal sources of protein and fat increases mortality, with a hazard ratio of 1.1, although there were criticisms on the methods [107]. A 2003 meta-analysis that included randomized controlled trials found that "low-carbo-hydrate, non-energy-restricted diets, appear to be at least as effective as low-fat, energy-restricted diets in inducing weight loss for up to 1 year [108]. Gardner *et al.* [109] compared the 4 special diet including the Atkins (a low-carbohydrate), Zone (by Barry Sears PhD, 40% carbohydrates, 30% protein, and 30% fats), Ornish (very low fat diet), and LEARN diets (55% to 60% energy from carbohydrate and less than 10% energy from saturated fat) to evaluate the effects of weight loss, metabolic effects and the risk over 1 year in 311 obese, non-diabetic, premenopausal women with randomized design. Weight loss was significantly greater for women in the Atkins diet group (low carbohydrate) compared with the other 3 diet groups at 12 months, and weight loss in the other 3 groups were similar, but at 12 months, secondary outcomes for the Atkins group were more favorable metabolic effects than the other diet groups. While questions remain about long-term effects and mechanisms, a low-carbohydrate, high-protein, high-fat diet may be considered a feasible alternative recommendation for weight loss. However, some investigators suggested that that one of the reasons people lose weight on low carbohydrate diet is related to the phenomenon of spontaneous reduction in food intake [110].

Previously, in routine practice a reduced-carbohydrate, higher protein diet was recommended approach to reducing the risk of cardiovascular disease and type 2 diabetes [111]. In 2004, the American Diabetes Association (ADA) affirmed its acceptance of carbohydrate-controlled diets as an effective treatment for short-term (up to one year) weight loss among obese people suffering from type 2 diabetes [112]. And the American Diabetes Association (ADA) revised their *"Nutrition Recommendations and Interventions for Diabetes in 2008"* to acknowledge low-carbohydrate diets as a legitimate weight-loss plan [113]. The recommendation, however, fell short of endorsing low-carbohydrate diets as a long-term health plan nor do they give any preference to these diets. On the other hand, the official statement from the American Heart Association (AHA) regarding these diets states categorically that the association doesn't recommend high-protein diets [35]. A science advisory from the AHA further states the association's belief that these diets are associated with increased risk for coronary heart disease [114, 115]. The AHA has been one of the most adamant opponents of low-carbohydrate diets. The American Heart Association supported low-fat and low-saturated-fat diets, but that a low-carbohydrate diet could not potentially meet AHA guidelines.

ii.   Low fat diet

Recently, the effectiveness of low-fat high- protein and low-fat high-carbohydrate dietary advice on weight loss were compared using group-based interventions, among overweight people with type 2 diabetes. However, in a 'real-world' setting, prescription of an energy-reduced low-fat diet, with either increased protein or carbohydrate, results in similar modest losses in weight, waist circumference and metabolic benefits over 2 years [116].

Ebbeling *et al.* [117] investigated the effect of dietary composition on energy expenditure during weight-loss maintenance among the 3 different diet groups (low-fat diet, low-glycemic index diet, and very low carbohydrate diet) with a controlled 3-way crossover design involving 21 overweight and obese young adults each for 4 weeks. Resting energy expenditure (REE), total energy expenditure (TEE), hormone levels, and metabolic syndrome components at pre-weight-loss were compared. Decreases in REE and TEE following 10% or 15% weight loss were greatest with the low-fat diet, intermediate with the low-glycemic index diet, and least with the very low-carbohydrate diet, but metabolic or hormonal parameters were similar between 3 groups.

iii.   Low glycemic index

The concept of the glycemic index was developed about 1981 by Dr. David Jenkins to account for variances in speed of digestion of carbohydrates. This concept classifies foods according to the rapidity of their effect on blood sugar levels – with fast digesting simple carbohydrates causing a sharper increase and slower digesting complex carbohydrates such as whole grains a slower one. The concept has been extended to include amount of carbohydrate actually absorbed as well, despite differences in glycemic index [118].

7.2. Pharmacological treatments for type 2 diabetes

If the individuals failed to improve glucose levels or HbA1c, pharmacological therapy is required. The first-line oral agents should minimize the degree of insulin resistance and suppress hepatic glucose production rather than increase plasma insulin concentrations. The decision to include thiazolidinediones (TZDs) and metformin as first-line therapy draws from the algorithm proposed by Wyne *et al.* [118]. Garber *et al.* [120] reported that Initial combination treatment with glyburide/metformin tablets produces greater improvements in glycemic control than either glyburide or metformin monotherapy.

The goal for glucose control is shown in Table 2 [11, 121]. Stimulating insulin secretion and minimizing insulin resistance both have the potential to bring a patient to goal, but it is theorized that bringing a patient to goal by reducing insulin resistance is more likely to reduce the macro-vascular complications and cardiovascular risks.

Based on several long-term, prospective studies which showed the significant reductions in cardiovascular risks associated with diabetes, the American Diabetes Association and American Association of Clinical Endocrinologists set forth standards and guidelines for the medical management of diabetes [11]. The recommendations clearly outline a multifactorial plan for managing diabetes and reducing complications [11], but they do not provide specific recommendations for selection and titration of pharmacological treatment. Pharmacological treatment for glucose control aims to reduce cardiovascular risk and to delay diabetic complications.

Glycemic control	A1C goal of < 7.0%	Measure every 3 months
Blood pressure control	< 130/80 mmHg	Every visit
Lipid control LDL	< 70 mg/dl†	Measure yearly or
Triglycerides	< 150 mg/dl	more frequently
HDL	> 45 mg/dl if	goals are not met
Urine protein Microalbuminuria	<30 mg/24 hours	Measure yearly

*American Diabetes Association Standards of medical care for patients with diabetesmellitus. *Diabetes Care* 26 (Suppl.):S33–S50, 2003.

†National Cholesterol Education Program: Implications of clinical trials for the ATP

Table 2. Diabetes Control Goals (by American Diabetes Association) Goals Endpoints Assessment

Pharmacological treatment for the management of obesity is primarily aimed at weight loss, weight loss maintenance and cardiovascular risk reduction. Anti-obesity agents decrease appetite, reduce absorption of fat or increase energy expenditure. Recently, anti-obesity drugs such as orlistat, sibtramine and rimonabant have been developed and placed on markets, however, the latter two were withdrawn from markets in the United States, Europe and Australia due to serious adverse events including psychiatric and cardiovascular related concerns. Recently, contrave, a combination of two approved drugs of bupropion and naltrexone, completed Phase III trials with significant weight loss and was approved by FDA in 2010, but subsequently the FDA declined to approve contrave due to serious cardiovascular adverse events in 2011 [122]. A contrave cardiovascular outcome trial, called "Light Study", is ongoing and is expected to be completed by the first quarter of 2013. Importantly, obesity is, at least, in part, determined by genetic backgrounds [123], suggesting that a genetic approach to limiting obesity may find a place in the future.

7.3. Bariatric surgery

Gastric bypass and adjustable gastric banding are the two most commonly performed bariatric procedures for the treatment of morbid obesity or obesity which is resistant to lifestyle modification such as a low caloric diet plus exercise. Multiple mechanisms contribute to the improved glucose metabolism seen after bariatric surgery, including caloric restriction, changes in the enteroinsular axis, alterations in the adipoinsular axis, release of nutrient-stimulated hormones from endocrine organs, stimulation from the nervous system, and psychosocial aspects including a dramatic improvement in quality of life [124]. Dixon *et al.* [86, 125] showed that gastric banding induced significant weight loss and resulted in better glucose control and less need for diabetes medication than conventional approaches to weight loss and diabetes control in a randomized controlled study in obese subjects with recently diagnosed type 2 diabetes. Koshy *et al.*[124] and other investigators [126, 127] compared the effects on weight loss, mortality, morbidity and changes in quality of life in subjects with either gastric bypass or gastric banding. The percent of excess weight loss at 4 years was higher in the gastric bypass group compared to the gastric banding group. Postoperative HOMA-IR correlated with % weight loss [126]. Concurrent with restoration of insulin sensitivity and decreases in plasma leptin were dramatic decreases in skeletal muscle at 3 and 9 months after gastric banding and a significant decrease in peroxisome proliferation activated receptor-alpha-regulated genes at 9 months. Gumbs *et al.* [128] speculated that a decrease in fat mass after bariatric surgery significantly affected circulating adipocytokines, which favourably influenced insulin resistance. Improvements in glucose metabolism and insulin resistance following bariatric surgery occur, in the short-term from decreased stimulation of the entero-insular axis by restricted calorie intake and in the long-term by decreased release of adipocytokines due to reduced fat mass. Leptin levels drop and adiponectin levels rise following laparoscopic adjustable gastric banding and gastric bypass. These changes correlate with weight loss and improvement in insulin sensitivity [128].

All forms of weight loss surgery lead to calorie restriction, weight loss, decrease in fat mass, and improvement in insulin resistance, type 2 diabetes mellitus, obesity and obesity-related hypertension [127]. Left ventricular relaxation impairment, assessed by tissue Doppler imaging, normalized 9 months after surgery [129]. Laparoscopic gastric bypass and gastric banding are both safe and effective approaches for the treatment of morbid obesity, but gastric bypass surgery seems to exert a better early weight loss and more rapid ameliorative effects on insulin resistance and adipocytokines, muscle metabolism and left ventricular function.

8. Conclusion

The prevalence of diabetes, especially type 2 diabetes and hypertension are significantly increased due, at least in part, to the increased prevalence of obesity. Type 2 diabetes is frequently associated with obesity, and is an important risk factor for cardiovascular morbidity and mortality and cardiac- and renal complications. Type 2 diabetes, hypertension and obesity are characterized by stimulation of the renin-angiotensin-aldosterone system (RAAS), elevated sympathetic activity and insulin resistance. Importantly, these characteristics, themselves, confer cardiovascular risk. Therefore, treatments for type 2 diabetes should be selected from favourable effects on stimulated RAAS, elevated sympathetic nervous system activity, insulin and leptin resistance.

Weight loss is recommended as the first line of treatment for type 2 diabetes and hypertension associated with type 2 diabetes in obesity. Lifestyle modification such as a caloric restricted diet, reducing sedentary behaviour and increases in exercise form the basis of all therapy. Weight loss treated with lifestyle modification including calorie restriction and/or exercise causes normalization of stimulated RAAS, sympathetic activation, insulin resistance, and hyperleptinemia. Recently, Masuo *et al.* [5] and Straznicky *et al.* [4] have shown that low caloric diet and exercise have different effects on insulin resistance, the RAAS, and sympathetic nervous activity in obese hypertensive subjects, even though similar weight loss was observed. Exercise had stronger effects on normalizing the RAAS stimulation, sympathetic activation and insulin resistance compared to diet only. The observations demonstrate that a combination therapy for weight loss with a low caloric diet and exercise is recommended for weight loss due to stronger suppression of insulin resistance and sympathetic activation, which both, themselves, are known as risk factors for cardiovascular events. Although few studies have observed changes in body weight, blood pressure, RAAS, sympathetic nervous activity, insulin resistance and leptin resistance over a long duration such as more than 2 years, Masuo et al. [6] observed more than 30% individuals who initially succeeded to significantly lose weight, had rebound weight gain over 2 years. Maintenance of weight loss is another key factor to delay and prevent type 2 diabetes and to reduce cardiovascular risks in type 2 diabetes in obesity.

In addition, special diets such as a low carbohydrate diet were reported as beneficial on weight loss previously, but it might cause an increase in cardiac risk. The official statement from American Heart Association reported that high-protein diet and low carbohydrate diet are not recommended diets due to increases in cardiovascular risk.

Gastric bypass and adjustable gastric banding are the two most commonly performed bariatric procedures for the treatment of morbid obesity or obesity which is resistant to lifestyle modification such as a low caloric diet plus exercise. Weight loss by bariatric surgery leads to improvement or normalization of glucose metabolisms from multiple mechanisms including caloric restriction, changes in the enteroinsular axis, alterations in the adipoinsular axis, release of nutrient-stimulated hormones from endocrine organs, stimulation from the nervous system, and psychosocial aspects including a dramatic improvement in quality of life.

Understanding the mechanisms underlying type 2 diabetes in obesity may help to achieve weight loss and maintenance of weight loss and resultant better control on type 2 diabetes, and delay and prevent the onset of type 2 diabetes or reduce complications.

This review provides information regarding, i) the importance of lifestyle medication on type 2 diabetes in obesity, ii) different effects of lifestyle modifications on weight loss and neurohormonal parameters between diet and exercise, and iii) the mode of weight loss and how it influences different physiological pathways. Different mechanisms may contribute to control in blood glucose levels and blood pressure and cardiovascular risks associated with weight loss with the relevant physiological mechanisms at play being dependent on the mode of weight loss.

Author details

Kazuko Masuo[1,2]

1 Nucleus Network Ltd., Baker IDI Heart & Diabetes Institute, Australia

2 Human Neurotransmitters Laboratory, Baker IDI Heart & Diabetes Institute, Australia

References

[1] Year Book Australia, 2012, 1301.0. Australian Bureau of Statistics. (24/5/2012)

[2] Mokdad AH, Ford ES, Bowman BA, Dietz WH, Vinicor F, Bales VS, Marks JS. Prevalence of obesity, diabetes, and obesity-related health risk factors, 2001. JAMA, 2003; 289(1): 76-79.

[3] The ORIGIN Trial Investigators. Basal insulin and cardiovascular and other outcomes in dysglycemia. N Engl J Med 2012;367(4):319-28. doi: 10.1056/ NEJMoa1203858. Epub 2012 Jun 11.

[4] Straznicky NE, Grima MT, Eikelis N, et al. The effects of weight loss versus weight loss maintenance on sympathetic nervous system activity and metabolic syndrome components. J Clin Endocrinol Metab. 2011; 96(3): E503-8.

[5] Masuo K, Rakugi H, Ogihara T, Lambert GW. Different mechanisms in weight loss-induced blood pressure reduction between a calorie-restricted diet and exercise. Hypertens Res. 2012; 35(1): 41-7. doi: 10.1038/hr.2011.134.

[6] Masuo K, Katsuya T, Kawaguchi H, Fu Y, Rakugi H, Ogihara T, Tuck ML. Rebound weight gain as associated with high plasma norepinephrine levels that are mediated through polymorphisms in the beta2-adrenoceptor. Am J Hypertens. 2005; 18(11): 1508-16.

[7] Kumar AA, Palamaner Subash Shantha G, Kahan S, Samson RJ, Boddu ND, Cheskin LJ. Intentional weight loss and dose reductions of anti-diabetic medications--a retrospective cohort study. PLoS One. 2012; 7(2): e32395.

[8] Masuo K, Mikami H, Ogihara T, Tuck ML. Weight reduction and pharmacologic treatment in obese hypertensives. Am J Hypertens. 2001; 14(6 Pt 1): 530-8.

[9] merican Diabetes Association. Diagnosis and classification of diabetes mellitus. Diabetes Care. 2012; 35 Suppl 1: S64-71.

[10] Kumar H, Mishra M, Bajpai S, Pokhria D, Arya AK, Singh RK, Tripathi K. Correlation of insulin resistance, beta cell function and insulin sensitivity with serum sFas and sFasL in newly diagnosed type 2 diabetes. Acta Diabetol. 2011 Jun 22. [Epub ahead of print].

[11] American Diabetes Association. Executive Summary: Standards of Medical Care in Diabetes—2012. Diabetes Care 2012; 35: S4-S10; doi:10.2337/dc12-s004.

[12] Eckert K. Impact of physical activity and bodyweight on health-related quality of life in people with type 2 diabetes. Diabetes Metab Syndr Obes. 2012; 5: 303-11.

[13] Diabetes Australia website, http://www.diabetesaustralia.com.au/living-with-diabetes/gestational-diabetes/./ Last Update: 21/06/2012. (accessed 15 November 2012).

[14] National Diabetes Statistics, 2011. National Institute of Diabetes and Digestive and Kidney Diseases website. www.diabetes.niddk.nih.gov/dm/pubs/statistics/index.aspx. Updated February 2011. (accessed on 15 November 2012).

[15] Katon J, Maynard C, Reiber G. Attempts at weight loss in U.S. women with and without a history of gestational diabetes mellitus. Womens Health Issues. 2012 Sep; 22(5):e447-53. doi: 10.1016/j.whi.2012.07.004.(accessed 10 November 2012).

[16] O'Keeffe M, St-Onge MP. Sleep duration and disorders in pregnancy: implications for glucose metabolism and pregnancy outcomes. Int J Obes (Lond). 2012 Sep 4. doi: 10.1038/ijo.2012.142.

[17] Carulli L, Rondinella S, Lombardini S, Canedi I, Loria P, Carulli N. Review article: Duiabetes, genetic and ethnicity. Alimentary Pharmacology & Therapeutics. 2005; 22 Suppl 2: 16-9.

[18] Meetoo D, McGovern P, Safadi R. An epidemiological overview of diabetes across the world. British Journal of Nursing. 2007; 16(16): 1002-7.

[19] Wold S, Roglic G, Green A, Sicree R, King H. Global prevalence of diabetes: estimates for the year 2000 and projections for 2030. Diabetes Care. 2004; 27 (5): 1047-1055.

[20] Centers for Diseases Control and Prevention (CDC). National Diabetes Fact Sheet, 2011. 2011. www.cdc.gov/diabetes/pubs/pdf/ndfs_2011.pdf

[21] Cali AM, Caprio S. Prediabetes and type 2 diabetes in youth: an emerging epidemic disease? Curr Opin Endocrinol Diabetes Obes. 2008; 15(2):123-7.

[22] Khalil AC, Roussel R, Mohammedi K, Danchin N, Marre M. Cause-specific mortality in diabetes: recent changes in trend mortality. Eur J Prev Cardiol. 2012; 19(3): 374-81.

[23] Abate N, Chandalia M. Ethnicity and type 2 diabetes: focus on Asian Indians. J Diabetes Complicat. 2001; 15(6): 320-7.

[24] Christian P, Sterwart CP. Maternal micronutrient deficiency, fetal development, and the risk of chronic disease. J Nutr. 2010; 140(3): 437-45.

[25] Latry P, Molimard M, Dedieu B, Couffinhal T, Bégaud B, Martin-Latry K. Adherence with statins in a real-life setting is better when associated cardiovascular risk factors increase: a cohort study. BMC Cardiovasc Disord. 2011 Jul 26;11:46. doi: 10.1186/1471-2261-11-46.

[26] Lardizabal JA, Deedwania PC. Benefits of statin therapy and compliance in high risk cardiovascular patients. Vasc Health Risk Manag. 2010; 6: 843–853.

[27] Narla V, Blaha MJ, Blumenthal RS, Michos ED. The JUPITER and AURORA clinical trials for rosuvastatin in special primary prevention populations: perspectives, outcomes, and consequences. Vasc Health Risk Manag. 2009; 5: 1033–1042.

[28] Tonelli M, Lloyd A, Clement F, et al. for the Alberta Kidney Disease Network. Efficacy of statins for primary prevention in people at low cardiovascular risk: a meta-analysis;. CMAJ. 2011; 183(16): e1189–e1202.

[29] Yang EY, Nambi V, Tang Z, Virani SS, Boerwinkle E,Hoogeveen RC, et al. Clinical implications of JUPITER in a United States population: insights from the Atherosclerosis Risk in Communities (ARIC) Study. J Am Coll Cardiol. 2009; 54(25): 2388–2395.

[30] Culver AL, Ockene IS, Balasubramanian R, Olendzki BC, Sepavich DM, Wactawski-Wende J, et al. Statin use and risk of diabetes mellitus in postmenopausal women in the Women's Health Initiative.. Arch Intern Med. 2012; 172(2): 144-52.

[31] Coleman CI, Reinhart K, Kluger J, White CM. The effect of statins on the development of new-onset type 2 diabetes: a meta-analysis of randomized controlled trials. Curr Med Res Opin. 2008; 24(5): 1359-62.

[32] Sattar N, Preiss D, Murray HM, Welsh P, Buckley BM, de Craen AJ, et al. Statins and risk of incident diabetes: a collaborative meta-analysis of randomised statin trials. Lancet. 2010; 375(9716): 735-42.

[33] Preiss D, Seshasai SR, Welsh P, Murphy SA, Ho JE, Waters DD, et al. Risk of incident diabetes with intensive-dose compared with moderate-dose statin therapy: a meta-analysis.. JAMA; 305(24): 2556-64.

[34] McEvoy JW. Statin therapy dose and risk of new-onset diabetes. JAMA. 2011; 306(12):1325-6.

[35] American Heart Association statement on high-protein, low-carbohydrate diet study presented at scientific sessions. American Heart Association press release, Nov 19, 2012.

[36] Filippatos TD. A Review of Time Courses and Predictors of Lipid Changes with Fenofibric Acid-Statin Combination. Cardiovasc Drugs Ther. 2012 June; 26(3): 245–255.

[37] Uchechukwu K. Sampson, MacRae F. Linton, Sergio Fazio. Are statins diabetogenic? Curr Opin Cardiol. 2011; 26(4): 342–347.

[38] The ACCORD Study Group. Effects of Combination Lipid Therapy in Type 2 Diabetes Mellitus. N Engl J Med. 2010; 362(17): 1563-74.

[39] Tenenbaum A, Fisman EZ. Balanced pan-PPAR activator bezafibrate in combination with statin: comprehensive lipids control and diabetes prevention? Cardiovasc Diabetes. 2012; 11(1):140.

[40] Carmena R, Betteridge DJ. Statins and diabetes. Semin Vas Med. 2004; 4 (4): 321-332.

[41] Heidmann C, Boeing H, Pischon T, Nothlings U, Joost HG, Schulze MB. Association of a diabetes risk score with risk of myocardial infarction, stroke, specific types of cancer, and mortality: a prospective study in the European Prospective Investigation

into Cancer and Nutrition (EPIC)-Potsdam cohort. Eur J Epidemiol. 2009; 24(6): 281-8.

[42] Preis SR, Hwang SJ, Coady S, Pencina MJ, D'Agostino RB Sr, Savage DJ, et al. Trends in all cause and cardiovascular disease mortality among women and men with and without diabetes mellitus in the Framingham Heart Study, 1950 to 2005. Circulation. 2009; 119(13): 1728-35.

[43] Lutufo PA, Gaziano M, Chae CU, Ajani UA, Moreno-John G, Buring JE, et al. Diabetes and all-cause and coronary heart disease mortality among US male physicians. Arch Intern Med. 2001; 161(2): 242-7.

[44] Kanaya AM, Grady D, Barrett-Connor E. Explaining the sex difference in coronary heart disease mortality among patients with type 2 diabetes mellitus: a meta-analysis. Arch Intern Med. 2002; 162(15): 1737-45.

[45] Young LH, Wackers FJ, Chyun DA, Davay JA, Barrett EJ, Taillefer R, et al. for DIAD Investigators. Cardiac outcomes after screening for asymptomatic coronary artery disease in patients with type 2 diabetes: the DIAD study: a randomized controlled trial. JAMA. 2009; 301(15): 1547-55.

[46] Morrison JA, Glueck CJ, Horn PS, Schreiber GH, Wang P. Pre-teen insulin resistance patients weight gain, impaired fasting glucose, and type 2 diabetes at age 18-19: a 10-y prospective study of black and white girls. Am J Clin Nutr. 2008; 88(3): 778-88.

[47] Koska J, Ortega E, Bogardus C, Krakoff J, Bunt JC. The effect of insulin on net lipid oxidation predicts worsen of insulin resistance and development of type 2 diabetes mellitus. Am J Physiol Endocrinol Metab. 2007; 293(1): 1264-1269.

[48] Rossing P, Hougaard P, Parving HH. Risk factors for development of incipient and overt diabetic nephropathy in type 1 diabetic patients: a 10-year prospective observational study. Diabetes Care. 2002; 25(5): 859-864.

[49] Cho E, RimmEB, Stampfer MJ, Willett WC, Hu FB. The impact of diabetes mellitus and prior myocardial infarction on mortality from all causes and from coronary heart disease in men. J Am Coll Cardiol. 2002; 40(5): 954-60.

[50] Iglseder B, Cip P, Malaimare L, Ladurner G, Paulweber B. The metabolic syndrome is a stronger risk factor for early carotid atherosclerosis in women than in men. Stroke. 2005; 36(6): 1212-7.

[51] Kawamoto R, Tomita H, Ohtsuka N, Inoue A, Kamitani A. Metabolic syndrome, diabetes and subclinical atherosclerosis as assessed by carotid intima-media thickness. J Atheroscler Thromb. 2007; 14(2): 78-85.

[52] Bertoni A, Wong ND, Shea S, et al. Insulin resistance, metabolic syndrome, and subclinical atherosclerosis. The Multi-Ethnic Study of Atheroclerosis (MESA). Diabetes Care. 2007; 30: 2951-6.

[53] Held C, Gerstein HC, Yusuf S, Ma S, Liu K, Preethi S, et al. for the ONTARGET/ TRANSCEND investigators. Glucose levels predict hospitalization for congestive heart failure in patients at high cardiovascular risk. Circulation. 2007; 115(11): 1371-5.

[54] Schulze MB, Hoffmann K, Boeing H, Linseisen J, Rothmann S, Mohilg M, et al. An accurate risk score based on anthropometric, dietary, and lifestyle factors to predict the development of type 2 diabetes. Diabetes Care. 2007; 30(3): 510-15.

[55] Morrison JA, Glueck CJ, Umar M, Daniels S, Dolan LM, Wang P. Hyperinsulinemia and metabolic syndrome at mean age of 10 years in black and white schoolgirls and development of impaired fasting glucose and type 2 diabetes mellitus by mean age of 24 years. Metabolism. 2011; 60(1): 24-31.

[56] Masuo K. Obesity-related hypertension: Role of sympathetic nervous system, insulin, and leptin. Curr Hypertens Rep. 2002; 4(2): 112-8.

[57] Esler M, Straznicky N, Eikelis N, Masuo K, Lambert G, Lambert E. Mechanism of sympathetic activation in obesity-related hypertension. Hypertension. 2006; 48(5): 787-96.

[58] Masuo k, Mikami H, Ogihara T, Tuck ML. Weight gain-induced blood pressure elevation. Hypertension. 2000; 35(5): 1135-40.

[59] Gentile CL, Orr JS, Davy BM, Davy KP. Modest weight gain is associated with sympathetic neural activation in nonobese humans. Am J Physiol Regul Interg Comp Phisiol. 2007; 292(5); R1834-38.

[60] Barnes MJ, Lapanowski K, Conley A, Rafols JA, Jen KL, Dunbar JC. High fat feeding is associated with increased blood pressure, sympathetic nerve activity and hypothalamic mu opioid receptors. Brain Res Bull. 2003; 61(5): 511-9.

[61] Anderson B, Elam M, Wallin BG, Bjorntorp P, Anderson OK. Effect of energy-restricted diet on sympathetic muscle nerve activity in obese women. Hypertension. 1991; 18(6): 783-9.

[62] Straznicky NE, Lambert EA, Lambert GW, Masuo K, Esler MD, Nestle PJ. Effects of dietary weight loss on sympathetic activity and cardiac risk factors associated with the metabolic syndrome. J Clin Endocrinol Met. 2005; 90(11): 5998-6005.

[63] Tuck ML, Sowers JR, Dornfeld L, Whitfield L, Maxwell M. Reductions in plasma catecholamines and blood pressure during weight loss in obese subjects. Acta Endocrinol (Copenh). 1983; 102(2): 252-7.

[64] Grassi G, Seravalle G, Colombo M, Bolla G, Cattaneo BM, Cavagnini F, et al. Body weight reduction, sympathetic nerve traffic, and arterial baroreflex in obese normotensive humans. Circulation. 1998; 97(20): 2037-2042.

[65] Masuo K, Katsuya T, Ogihara T, Tuck ML. Acute hyperinsulinemia reduces plasma leptin levels in insulin sensitive men. Am J Hypertens. 2005; 18(2 Pt 1): 235-43.

[66] Huggett RJ, Scott EM, Gilbey SG, Stoker JB, Mackintosh AF, Mary DASG. Impact of type 2 diabetes mellitus on sympathetic neural mechanisms in hypertension. Circulation. 2003; 108(25): 3097-3101.

[67] Staznicky NE, Lambert GW, Masuo K, et al. Blunted sympathetic neural response to oral glucose in obese subjects with the insulin-resistant metabolic syndrome. Am J Clin Nutr. 2009; 89: 27-36.

[68] Straznicky NE, Grima MT, Sari CI, Eikelis N, Lambert EA, Nestel PJ, et al. Neuroadrenergic dysfunction along the diabetes continuum: a comparative study in obese metabolic syndrome subjects. Diabetes. 2012; 61(10): 2506-16.

[69] Takatori S, Zamami Y, Mio M, Kurosaki Y, Kawasaki H. Chronic hyperinsulinemia enhances adrenergic vasoconstriction and decreases calcitonin gene-related peptide-containing nerve-mediated vasodilation in pithed rats. Hypertens Res. 2006; 29(5): 361-368.

[70] Zamami Y, Takatori S, Yamawaki K, Miyashita S, Mio M, Kitamura Y, Kawasaki H. Acute hyperglycemia and hyperinsulinemia enhance adrenergic vasoconstriction and decrease calcitonin gene-related peptide-containing nerve-mediated vasodilation in pithed rats. Hypertens Res. 2008(5); 31: 1033-1044.

[71] Gudbjornsdottir S, Elam M, Sellgren J, Anderson EA. Insulin increases forearm vascular resistance in obese, insulin-resistant hypertensives. J Hypertens. 1996; 14(1): 91-7.

[72] van Veen S, Frolich M, Chang PC. Acute hyperglycemia in the forearm induces vasodilation that is not modified by hyperinsulinemia. J Human Hypertens. 1999; 13(4): 263-68.

[73] Thethi T, Kamiyama M, Kobori H. The link between the renin-angiotensin-aldosterone system and renal injury in obesity and the metabolic syndrome. Curr Hypertens Rep. 2012; 14(2): 160-9.

[74] Maser RE, Lenhard MJ, Kolm P, Edwards DG. Direct renin inhibition improves parasympathetic function in diabetes. Diabetes Obes Metab. 2013; 15(1): 28-34. 2012 Jul 27. doi: 10.1111/j.1463-1326.2012.01669.x.

[75] Kosaka K, Noda M, Kuzuya T. Prevention of type 2 diabetes by lifestyle intervention: a Japanese trial in IGT males. Diabetes Res Clin Pract. 2005; 67(2): 152-62.

[76] Masuo K, Rakugi H, Ogihara T, Esler MD, Lambert GW. Effects of weight loss on renal function in overweight Japanese men. Hypertens Res. 2011; 34(8): 915-21.

[77] Masuo K, Rakugi H, Ogihara T, Esler MD, Lambert GW. Cardiovascular and renal complications of type 2 diabetes in obesity: role of sympathetic nerve activity and insulin resistance. Curr Diabetes Rev. 2010; 6(2): 58-67.

[78] Straznicky NE, Grima MT, Lambert EA, et al. Exercise augments weight loss induced improvement in renal function in obese metabolic syndrome individuals. J Hypertens. 2011; 29(3): 553-64

[79] Masuo K, Lambert GW, Esler MD, Rakugi H, Ogihara T, Schlaich MP. The role of sympathetic nervous activity in renal injury and end-stage renal disease. Hypertens Res. 2010; 33(6): 521-8.

[80] Masuo K, Rakugi H, Ogihara T, Tuck ML. β1 (Arg389Gly, Ser49Gly)- and β2 (Arg16Gly)-adrenoceptor polymorphisms are related to left ventricular hypertrophy in middle-aged, nonobese,1 normotensive men, but through different mechanisms. Circulation. 2008; 18 (119) Suppl 2: S1154.

[81] Orchard TJ, Temprosa M, Goldberg R, Haffner S, Ratner R, Marcovina S, Fowler S. The effect of metformin and intensive lifestyle intervention on the metabolic syndrome: The Diabetes Prevention Program randomized trial. Ann Intern Med. 2005; 142(8): 611-619.

[82] Anderssen SA, Carroll S, Urdal P, Holme I. Combined diet and exercise intervention reverses the metabolic syndrome in middle-aged males: results from the Oslo Diet and Exercise Study. Scand J Med Sci Sports. 2007; 17(6): 687-95.

[83] Allison DB, Zannolli R, Faith MS, Heo M, Piethobelli A, Vanltallie TB, et al. Weight loss increases and fat loss decreases all-cause mortality rate: results from two independent cohort studies. Int J Obes Relat Metab Disord. 1999; 23(6): 603-11.

[84] Poobalan AS, Aucott LS, Smith WCS, Avenell A, Jung R, Broom J. Long-term weight loss effects on all cause mortality in overweight/obese populations. Obes Rev. 2007; 8(6): 503-13.

[85] Sjostrom L, Narbro K, Sjostrom CD, Karason K, Larsson B, Nedei H, et al. Effects of bariatric surgery on mortality in Swedish obese subjects. N Engl J Med. 2007; 357(8): 741-52.

[86] Dixon JB, O'Brien PE, Playfair J, Chapman L, Schachter LM, Skiner S, et al. Adjustable gastric banding and conventional therapy for type 2 diabetes: a randomized controlled trial. JAMA. 2008; 299(3): 316-23.

[87] Sierra-Johnson J, Romeo-Corral A, Somers VK, Lopez-Jimenez F, Thomas RJ, Squires RW, Allison TG. Prognostic importance of weight loss in patients with coronary heart disease regardless of initial body mass index. Eur J Cardiovasc Prev Rehabil. 2008; 15(3): 336-40.

[88] Masuo K, Mikami H, Ogihara T, Tuck ML. Differences in mechanisms between weight loss-sensitive and -resistant blood pressure reduction in obese subjects. Hypertens Res. 2001; 24(4):371-6.

[89] American Diabetes Association. Evidence-Based Nutrition Principles and Recommendations for the Treatment and Prevention of Diabetes and Related Complications. Diabetes Care January 2002; 25 (suppl 1): s50-s60.

[90] Toji C, Okamoto N, Kobayashi T, Furukawa Y, Tanaka S, Ueji K, et al. Effectiveness of diet versus exercise intervention on weight reduction in local Japanese residents. Environ Health Prev Med. 2012; 17(4): 332-40.

[91] Masuo K, Kawaguchi H, Mikami H, Ogihara T, Tuck ML. Serum uric acid and plasma norepinephrine concentrations predict subsequent weight gain and blood pressure elevation. Hypertension. 2003; 42(4): 474-80.

[92] Straznicky NE, Eikelis N, Nestel PJ,Dixon JB, Dawood T, Grima MT, et al. Baseline sympathetic nervous system activity predicts dietary weight loss in obese metabolic syndrome subjects. J Clin Endocrinol Metab. 2012; 97 (2): 605-13.

[93] Ribeiro MM, Silva AG, Santos NS, Guazzalle I, Mates LN, Tronbetta IC, et al. Diet and exercise training restore blood pressure and vasodilatory responses during physiological maneuvers in obese children. Circulation. 2005; 111(15): 1915-23

[94] Trombetta IC, Batalha LT, Rondon MU, et al. Gly16 + Glu27 beta2-adrenoceptor polymorphisms cause increased forearm blood flow responses to mental stress and handgrip in humans. J Appl Physiol. 2005; 98(3): 787-94

[95] Tonacio AC, Trombetta IC, Rondon MU, Laterza MC, Frazzatto E, Alves MJ, et al. Effects of diet and exercise training on neurovascular control during mental stress in obese women. Braz J Med Biol Res. 2006; 39(1): 53-62.

[96] Santarpia L, Contaldo F, Pasanisi F. Body composition changes after weight-loss interventions for overweight and obesity. Clin Nutr. 2013; 32(2): 157-61.

[97] Dumortier M, Brandou F, Perez-Martin A, Fedou C, Mercier J, Brun JF. Low intensity endurance exercise targeted for lipid oxidation improves body composition and insulin sensitivity in patients with the metabolic syndrome. Diabetes Metab. 2003; 29(5): 509-18.

[98] Poirier P, Pespres JP. Exercise in weight management of obesity. Cardio Clin. 2001; 19(3): 459-470.

[99] Skilton MR, Mikkilä V, Würtz P, Ala-Korpela M, Sim KA, Soinuinen P, et al. Fetal growth, omega-3 (n-3) fatty acids, and progression of subclinical atherosclerosis: preventing fetal origins of disease? The Cardiovascular Risk in Young Finns Study. Am J Clin Nutr. 2013; 97(1): 58-65.

[100] Mozaffarian D, Abdollahi M, Campos H, Houshiarrad A, Willett WC. Consumption of trans-fats and estimated effects on coronary heart disease in Iran. Eur J Clin Nutr. 2007; 61(8): 1004-10.

[101] Whitman SC, Rateri DL, Szilvassy SJ, Yokoyama W, Daugherty A. Depletion of natural killer cell function decreases atherosclerosis in low-density lipoprotein receptor null mice. Arterioscler Thromb Vasc Biol. 2004; 24(6): 1049-54.

[102] Teegala SM, Willett WC, Mozaffarian D. Consumption and health effects of trans fatty acids: a review. J AOAC Int. 2009; 92(5): 1250-7.

[103] Larsson SC, Virtamo J, Wolk A. Dietary fats and dietary cholesterol and risk of stroke in women. Atherosclerosis. 2012; 221(1): 282-6.

[104] Chowdhury R, Stevens S, Gorman D, Pan A, Wamakula S, Chowdhury S, et al. Association between fish consumption, long chain omega 3 fatty acids, and risk of cerebrovascular disease: systematic review and meta-analysis. BMJ. 2012 Oct 30;345:e6698. doi: 10.1136/bmj.e6698.

[105] Oh K, Hu FB, Manson JAE, Stampfer MJ, Willett WC. Dietary Fat Intake and Risk of Coronary Heart Disease in Women: 20 Years of Follow-up of the Nurses' Health Study. Am. J. Epidemiol. 2005; 161 (7): 672-9.

[106] Storlien LH, Baur LA, Kriketos AD, Pan DA, Cooney GJ, Jenkins AB, et al. Dietary fats and insulin action. Diabetologia. 1996; 39(6):621-31.

[107] Halton TL, Willett WC, Liu S, Manson JE, Albert CM, Rexrode K, et al. Low-Carbohydrate-Diet Score and the Risk of Coronary Heart Disease in Women. N Engl J Med. 2006; 355(19):1991-2002.

[108] Samaha FF, Iqbal N, Seshadri P, Chicano KL, Daily DA, McGrory J, Williams T, Williams M, et al. "A Low-Carbohydrate as Compared with a Low-Fat Diet in Severe Obesity". New England Journal of Medicine 2003; 348(21): 2074–81.

[109] Gardner CD, Kiazand A,Alhassan S, Kim S, Stafford RS, Balise RR, et al. Comparison of the Atkins, Zone, Ornish, and LEARN diets for change in weight and related risk factors among overweight premenopausal women: the A TO Z Weight Loss Study: a randomized trial. JAMA. 2007; 297(9): 969-77.

[110] Boden G, Sargrad K, Homko C, Mozzoli M, Stein TP, Effect of a low-carbohydrate diet on appetite, blood glucose levels, and insulin resistance in obese patients with type 2 diabetes. Annals of Internal Medicine. 2005, 142(6):403-411.

[111] McAuley KA, Hopkins CM, Smith KJ, McLay RT, Williams SM, Taylor RW, Mann JI. Comparison of high-fat and high-protein diets with a high-carbohydrate diet in insulin-resistant obese women. Diabetologia. 2005; 48(1): 8-16.

[112] Klein S, Sheard NF, Pi-Sunyer X,Daly A, Wylie-Rosett J, Kulkarni K, et al. Weight Management Through Lifestyle Modification for the Prevention and Management of Type 2 Diabetes: Rationale and Strategies. A statement of the American Diabetes Association, the North American Association for the Study of Obesity, and the American Society for Clinical Nutrition. Diabetes Care. 2004; 27(8): 2067-2073.

[113] Bantle JP, Wylie-Rosett J, Albright AL, APovian CM, Clark NG, Franz MJ, et al. American Diabetes Association (2008) Nutrition recommendations and interventions for diabetes: a position statement of the American Diabetes Association. Diabetes care. 2008; 31 Suppl: S61-S78.

[114] Kones R. Low-fat versus low-carbohydrate diets, weight loss, vascular health, and prevention of coronary artery disease: the evidence, the reality, the challenge, and the hope. Nutr Clin Pract. 2010; 25(5): 528-41

[115] St. Jeor ST, Howard BV, Prewitt E, Bovee V, Bazzarre T, Eckel RH. Dietary Protein and Weight Reduction: A Statement for Healthcare Professionals From the Nutrition Committee of the Council on Nutrition, Physical Activity, and Metabolism of the American Heart Association, American Heart Association, 2001.

[116] Krebs JD, Elley CR, Parry-Strong A, et al. The Diabetes Excess Weight Loss (DEWL) Trial: a randomised controlled trial of high-protein versus high-carbohydrate diets over 2 years in type 2 diabetes. Diabetologia. 2012; 55(4): 905-14.

[117] Ebbeling CB, Swain JF, Feldman HA, Wong WW, Hachey DL, Garcia-Lago E, Ludwig DS, Effects of dietary composition on energy expenditure during weight loss maintenance. JAMA. 2012; 307(24):2627-34.

[118] Jenkins DJA, Kendall CWC, Augustin LSA, Francrschi S, Hamidi M, Marchie A, et al. Glycemic index: overview of implications in health and disease. Am J Clin Nutr. 2002; 76(1):266S-73S.

[119] Wyne KL, Drexler AJ, Miller JL, Bell DS, Braunstein S, Nuckolls JG: Constructing an algorithm for managing type 2 diabetes: focus on the role of the thiazolidinediones. Postgrad Med. 2003 May; 8 Spec.63–72.

[120] Garber AJ, Larsen J, Schneider SH, Piper BA, Henry D. The Glyburide/Metformin Initial Therapy Study Group[1.] Simultaneous glyburide/metformin therapy is superior to component monotherapy as an initial pharmacological treatment for type 2 diabetes. Diabetes, Obesity and Metabolism. 2002; 4(3): 201-8.

[121] Chitre MM, Burke S. Treatment Algorithms and the Pharmacological Management of Type 2 Diabetes. Diabetes Spectrum. 2006;19(4):249-255.

[122] Greenway FL, Fujioka K, Plodkowski RA, Mudaliar S, Guttadauria M, Erickson J, Kim DD, Dunayevich E; COR-I Study Group. Effect of naltrexone plus bupropion on weight loss in overweight and obese adults (COR-I): a multicentre, randomised, double-blind, placebo-controlled, phase 3 trial. Lancet. 2010; 376(9741): 595-605.

[123] Heal DJ, Gosden J, Smith SL. What is the prognosis for new centrally-acting anti-obesity drugs? Neuropharmacology. 2012; 63(1): 132-46.

[124] Koshy AA, Babe AM, Brady MJ. Potential mechanisms by which bariatric surgery improves systemic metabolism. Transl Res. 2012. doi: 10.1016/j.trsl.2012.09.004.

[125] Dixon JB, Murphy DK, Segel JE, Finkelstein EA. Impact of laparoscopic adjustable gastric banding on type 2 diabetes. Obes Rev. 2012; 13(1): 57-67. doi: 10.1111/j. 1467-789X.2011.00928.x.

[126] Ballantyne GH, Wasielewski A, Saunders JK. The surgical treatment of type II diabetes mellitus: Changes in HOMA insulin resistance in the first year following laparoscopic Rou-en-Y gastric bypass (LRYGB) and laparoscopic adjustable gastric banding (LAGB). Obes Surg. 2009; 19(9): 1297-303. doi: 10.1007/s11695-009-9870-2.

[127] Trakhenbroit MA, Leichman JG, Algahim MF, Miller CC 3rd, Moody FG, Lux TR, Taegtmeyer H. Body weight, insulin resistance, and serum adipokine levels 2 years after 2 types of bariatric surgery. Am J Med. 2009; 122(5): 435-42. doi: 10.1016/ j.amjmed.2008.10.035.

[128] Gumbs AA, Modlin IM, Ballantyne GH. Changes in insulin resistance following bariatric surgery: role of caloric restriction and weight loss. Obes Surg. 2005; 15(4): 462-73.

[129] Leichman JG, Wilson EB, Scarborough T, Aguilar D, Miller CC 3rd, Yu S, Algahim MF, Reyes M, Moody FG, Taegtmeyer H. Dramatic reversal of derangements in muscle metabolism and left ventricular function after bariatric surgery. Am J Med. 2008; 121(11): 966-73. doi: 10.1016/j.amjmed.2008.06.033.

Chapter 3

Socio-Ecological Approach to Self-Management of Type 2 Diabetes: Physical Activity and Dietary Intervention

Rashid M. Ansari, John B. Dixon and
Colette J. Browning

Additional information is available at the end of the chapter

1. Introduction

The incidence of type 2 diabetes is increasing worldwide, resulting in large measure from the increasing prevalence of obesity (Yale, 2000). Diabetes mellitus is a pandemic disease and is one of the main threats to human health (Narayan, 2005). In 2003, 194 million people world-wide, ranging in age from 20 to 79 years, had diabetes. It is projected that this number will be increased by 72% to 333 million by 2025, and nearly 80% of these cases will be in the poorer industrialized countries (IDF, 2003).Type 2 diabetes is also a major public health problem in Pakistan as the middle-aged population in that country is overweight or obese, lack of physical activity, unhealthy food and eating habits exposing this population to a high risk of type 2 diabetes (Ansari, 2009). In the local context, prevalence of Type 2 diabetes in Pakistan for the year 2000 was 7.6 % (5.2 million populations) and for 2030 it will increase to around 15% (13.8 million populations) and as such Pakistan is ranked 7th on diabetes prevalence list (WHO, 2004). It was found by Jafar et al (2006) that on the age-specific prevalence of overweight and obesity, more than 40% of women and 30% of men aged 35–54 years were classified as overweight or obese.

Despite the high prevalence of diabetes and serious long term complications, there is still lack of established evidence-based guidelines for self-management (ADA, 2006) and translation of practice recommendations to care in Asian countries (Rayappa et al. 1998) and as well as in developed countries (Chin et al. 2000). Therefore, promoting an active lifestyle or regular exercise has become the highest public health priority in that country to overcome the onslaught of type 2 diabetes and in this context this project is very significant as it addresses this important problem of type 2 diabetes. There is a need for self-management approach for patients of type 2 diabetes and the assessment of quality of diabetes care in the community can help draw attention to the need for improving diabetes self-management and provide a benchmark for monitoring changes over time.

2. Brief literature review

A systematic review of the literature was carried out to cover socio-ecological approach to self-management of type 2 diabetes. Electronic databases were searched, including Cochrane library, Medline, Embase. References of all retrieved articles were checked for relevant studies.

The selection of studies was based on the following criteria:

Interventions: educational interventions compared with usual care, physical activity and diet interventions, behavioural intervention.

Participants: middle-aged population, aged 30-65 with poorly controlled type 2 diabetes.

Outcomes: Studies must report haemoglobin (HbA1c) or hypoglycemia episodes, diabetic complications, cardiovascular disease and quality of life.

Design: The studies related to socio-ecological approach to self-management of type 2 diabetes were included. The search key words were type 2 diabetes, socio-ecological intervention and self-management.

The literature survey revealed that diabetes self-management education is the cornerstone of diabetes care (Mensing et al. 2007). There are several studies indicated an association between diabetes self-management and improved diabetes knowledge and self-management behaviours and improved clinical outcomes (Norris et al. 2001; Philis-Tsimikas et al. 2004). However, authors of a meta-analysis of diabetes self-management programmes reported sharp declines in benefits within one month post intervention (Norris et al. 2001) suggesting that self-management interventions alone do not enable individuals to maintain behaviours changes. The improved outcomes were reported when diabetes self-management was carried out for a longer duration, community-based (CDC, 2001), included follow-up support (Norris et al. 2001), and provided culturally sensitive interventions (Philis-Tsimikas et al 2004; Brown et al. 2005), and addressed psychosocial issues (Mauldon et al. 2006; Norris et al. 2001).

In addition, the social interaction between the patients and doctors is of great significance. The patients of diabetes need to engage with a range of health professionals. Gaining knowledge of the patient's perspective builds on traditional models of physician-patient communication (Pendleton et al. 1984) provides greater clarity to the range of lay understandings that should be explored as a component of effective risk communication.

Fisher et al (2005) suggested that the quality clinical care and self management are compatible and dependent on each other and without sound care, individual's efforts may be misdirected and expert clinical care will fall far short of its potential, through patient failure to use prescribed medications to control his blood sugar or to implement its management plans (Fisher et al. 2005).

A framework for integrating the resources and supports for self-management with key components of clinical care was also provided by Wagner et al (1996) in their chronic care model. A number of studies have also suggested that patient understanding and beliefs about health and illness may be shaped by historical and local contexts (Macfarlane and Kelleher, 2002), whether respondents are thinking about health or behaviour in general or about their own (Blaxter, 1990; French et al. 2001), and personal experience and observation (Davison et al. 1991). The following figure 1 provides a conceptual framework of self-management of type 2 diabetes using the socio-ecological approach.

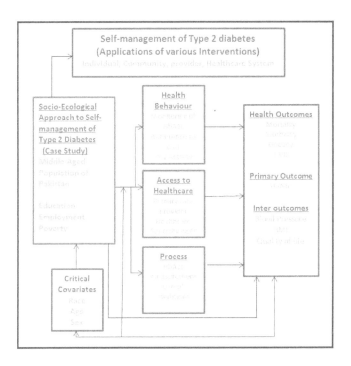

Figure 1. Conceptual framework of self-management of type 2 diabetes

3. Ecological approach to self-management

This case study would also demonstrate that the person is solely responsible to take care of his diabetes related problems and its management and therefore the issue of self-management becomes more important for those with chronic disease, where only the patient can be responsible for day to day care over the length of the illness (Lorig and Holman, 2003). It is generally agreed that self-management is required for control of chronic diseases and for prevention of disease complications; however, patients generally do not adhere to self-management recommendations (Sherbourne et al. 1992; Gochman, 1997; Glasgow and Eakin, 1998). The adherence to the recommendations and barriers are both problematic for "lifestyle" behaviour such as eating patterns and physical activity rather than medication adherence (Brown, 1990; Roter et al. 1998; Ansari, 2009). This is evident from the culture, tradition and life style behavior of the people of Pakistan that both the eating patterns and physical activity are posing a great deal of difficulties to middle-aged population with diabetes.

There is compelling evidence that higher levels of social support are related to better long-term self management and better health outcomes (Kaplan and Toshima, 1990; Uchino et al. 1996). There is also a significant relationship between support and health where support can be assessed from a variety of sources, including spouses, family, friends and neighbours (Dignam et al. 1986). The relationships between support and immunity (Cohen et al. 1997), health status and health behaviours (Glasgow and Toobert, 1988), mortality and quality of life (House et al. 1988; Glasgow et al. 1997) have also been reported in the literature. King et al (2010) has demonstrated that self-efficacy, problem solving, and social environment support are associated with diabetes self-management behaviours.

4. Health services in the local community

The health services in the community in Pakistan are not adequate and diabetes health management programme in the community health clinics does not provide enough help and support to the patients. Shortage of community doctors and expensive consultation with private doctors make the life of patients more difficult in terms of managing their diabetes in that region of Pakistan.

These clinics in Pakistan face special challenges to provide diabetes care to the poor patients as most of these clinics do not meet the evidence-based quality of care standards as compared to the targets established by the American Diabetes Association (ADA, 2000). Similar cases have been reported in several studies in diversified health care settings; including academic institutions (Peters et al. 1996), health maintenance organization (Miller and Hirsch, 1994), health centers (Chin et al. 2000) and medical providers (Chin et al. 1998) where substantial portion of diabetes care does not meet the evidence-based quality of standard care. Marshall et al (2000) have reported that community-based health clinics and their patients have fewer resources than the private clinics and the clinics often lack access to integrated delivery system, and their small size limits the financial feasibility of full-time teams devoted solely to diabetes care.

5. Interventions to improve health services in the community

The health services in the community can be improved by making use of on-going follow-up and support for the self-management of diabetes which has shown promising results (Norris et al. 2002). For the poor patients in that region of Pakistan where access to the community doctors is not easy and private doctors are not affordable, support may be provided through telephone calls (Weinberger et al. 1995) or the internet (McKay et al. 1998). It has been reported that telephone monitoring of patients, combined with nurse follow-up and tailored information has been shown to reach low income patients and helped them managed their blood sugar level and reduced levels of depression (Piette et al. 1999; Piette et al. 2000).

Another strategy to improve the health services in the community is the group visit to medical clinics by the patients of diabetes (Beck et al. 1997) in which all the patients in a particular category visit the physicians for general check-up including the educational and supportive discussions. Evaluation of this type of strategy has indicated impressive effects on glycosylated hemoglobin and other measures to usual care (Trento et al. 2001).

6. Self-management approach
in local context

In order to meet the main objective of this study, the socio-ecological approach to self-management of type 2 diabetes will be applied to middle-aged population of Pakistan using case study approach. The case study is most suitable as it integrates the skills and choices of individuals with the services and support they receive from (a) the social environment of family, friends, organizations and cultures (b) the physical and policy environments of neighbourhoods, communities and governments (Stokols, 1996). The self management from an ecological perspective requires access to a variety of resources, including services provided by professionals and support for the initiation and maintenance of healthy behaviours (Glasgow, 1995; Glasgow et al. 2000).

There is only one study conducted in Pakistan on diabetes knowledge, beliefs and practices among people with diabetes (Rafique et al. 2006). The study provided further evidence that there was a lack of information available to people with diabetes in Pakistan as the large population has never received any diabetes education at all (Rafique et al. 2006). Also, the study was conducted in an urban university hospital, where diabetes education may be more readily available as compared to rural areas where people have less access to information and will have even poorer diabetes perception and practices.

This case study would make a unique contribution to public health in the rural area of Pakistan. This will be first type detailed study of diabetes self-management among the population of Pakistan. It will address the issues and the ways in which diabetes in viewed and managed in that region. The study will also be useful for health care professionals suggesting that coping with diagnosis and living with diabetes is affected by a complex constellation of factors, including life circumstances, social support, gender roles and economy.

7. Aims and objectives

The main objective of this study is to examine the role of physical inactivity and obesity in the development of type 2 diabetes and its self-management in a middle-aged population living in rural area of Pakistan and to evaluate a lifestyle intervention (Physical Activity and Diet) in the management of type 2 diabetes. The study would use the qualitative health approach conducting one-on-one interviews with a sample of informants – patients of type 2 diabetes (n=210) and to explore patients perceptions and experiences of undertaking physical activity and eating behaviour as part of their diabetes self-management. In addition, the study would analyze how the health issue related to diabetes is viewed and addressed in the community and identify the barriers to diabetes care in community and healthcare clinics and would use the concepts of socio-ecological approach to self-management of type 2 diabetes.

This research protocol design addresses the lifestyle interventions for lowering hemoglobin (HbA1c) in this randomized controlled trial and determines whether the intervention of physical activity and diet in combination of usual medical care lowers HbA1c in patients with type 2 diabetes. These types of trials are critical and significant in determining if the culturally tailored interventions are effective in the practical world in which patients live as these patients with diabetes in sub-continent may have different characteristics than those in other western countries due to their eating of different foods and drinking habits.

In addition, this study will help to minimize the gap between the physician-patient under-standing and management of diabetes and to identify the barriers to self management of diabetes and quality of life. This study will contribute to improving the quality health care for diabetes in health clinics in that region and would recommend a multifactorial approach emphasizing patient education, improved training in behavioural change for providers, and enhanced delivery system (Chin et al. 2000). The understanding of people about diabetes and susceptibility to diabetes is linked to family, community and society and therefore, this study will impress upon the need to recognize that in developing strategies and interventions to address diabetes, self-care, family support, community education and community ownership are important (Weeramanthri et al. 2003; Wong et al. 2005).

Research Questions: The research questions have been formulated as follows:

1.   Will this study help to enhance the patient understanding of self-management of diabetes and will it minimize the gap between the physician-patient interactions?

2.   Will hemoglobin (HbA1c) improve after the 90 days trial of lifestyle interventions in patients with poorly controlled type 2 diabetes?

3.   Will physical activity and healthy diet lead to reducing the Body Mass Index (BMI) and consequently the risk of diabetes in patients of type 2 diabetes in that region?

Hypotheses: The following hypotheses are to be tested in this study:

1.   The lifestyle interventions (physical activity and diet) in patients with poorly controlled diabetes will lead to reduction of 1% hemoglobin (HbA1c) in 90 days trial. (HbA1c as Primary outcome variable)

2. The self-management of type 2 diabetes will reduce 5% weight in patients in 90 days trial and consequently the BMI (BMI as secondary outcome variable)

8. Justification of hypotheses

The justification of the first hypothesis stem from the fact that the clinical complications are significantly associated with glycemia (Stratton et al. 2000) and it has been reported that that each 1% reduction in hemoglobin (HbA1c) is associated with reductions in risk of 21% for any end point related to diabetes, 21% for deaths related to diabetes, 14% for myocardial infarction and 37% for microvascular complications (DCCT, 1996; UKPDS, 1998). The second hypothesis is related to Body Mass Index (BMI) and weight reduction which are measures of obesity and linked to the development of problems in glycemic control and are major risk factors for the development of cardiovascular disease (Michael, 2007).

9. Study design and sampling method

The patients will be recruited from the diabetic medical centre in rural area of Peshawar conducting the study of management of type 2 diabetes among the population aged 30-65 years. The eligibility of patients will be subjected to further screening if their records will not be found in the clinic database. The patients with diabetes having HbA1c >7.0% will be included in this study and patients having coexisting liver, kidney or thyroid disorder will be excluded from this study. The Word Health Organization (WHO, 2006) diabetes criteria will be followed in the selection of the patients with diabetes as indicated in Table 1.

Condition	2 hour glucose	Fasting glucose
	mmol/l(mg/dl)	mmol/l(mg/dl)
Normal	<7.8 (<140)	<6.1 (<110)
Impaired fasting glycaemia	<7.8 (<140)	≥ 6.1(≥110) & <7.0(<126)
Impaired glucose tolerance	≥7.8 (≥140)	<7.0 (<126)
Diabetes mellitus	≥11.1 (≥200)	≥7.0 (≥126)

Table 1. World Health Organization (WHO, 2006). Diabetes Criteria for patients

All the participants will adhere to their usual medications as recommended by their doctors. In order to assess the effectiveness of this intervention, it was advised not to modify the medications during this trial. In addition, participants will be advised not to take any other new treatments for the management of type 2 diabetes during this study. All participants will be contacted again after 90 days (3-months) to give their blood sample for HbA1c testing, their weight will be taken and BMI will be calculated.

10. Study population and randomization

Initially 325 patients with type 2 diabetes will be invited to pre-randomized interview, out of which only 210 patients will be included in the actual trial. For the purpose of this trial, it is expected that out of the 325 patients, 93 patients will not meet the inclusion criteria and 22 patients might refuse to participate in the trial. In that case, two hundred and ten (210) patients will agree to participate and will be required to sign informed consent documents at the clinic where they usually visit for their usual medical care for diabetes. Therefore, 105 patients will be randomized to intervention group (Physical Activity and Diet) and 105 to the control group (usual medical care). Figure 2 shows their progress during the randomized controlled trial. This RCT trial will not be double-blinded as the participants receiving the education on lifestyle modifications in the community and healthcare clinics would know that they are on the active intervention.

Once the randomization phase is completed, all patients will be instructed to follow-up the usual medical care for their diabetes for the duration of the 90 days trial. The patients will not be allowed to adjust their usual medications and follow their previous prescriptions recommended by their doctors. In addition, each patient will be asked to go for blood test for HbA1c on day 1 and then return to give blood sample after 90 days. In addition, participants will be advised not to take any other new treatments for the management of type 2 diabetes during the trial periods.

Those patients randomized to adhere to physical activity and diet (intervention group) will receive education, advice, and behaviour modification skills to help them to maintain a low fat diet, lose weight (goal of 5% weight loss) and moderate intensity physical activity such as brisk walking for 150 minutes/week. Those patients randomized to usual medical care (control group) will be instructed to take their normal medicines and follow-up with their doctor as per their normal schedule.

All participants will be contacted again after 90 days (3-months) to give their blood sample for HbA1c testing, their weight will be taken and BMI will be calculated. At that time, a questionnaire will be sent via e-mail to participants in intervention group to assess the progress of the physical activity and diet intervention and to control group to assess the progress of the treatment with normal medical care only.

11. Measurement

The factors which will be measured in this study are the physical activity of participants (an intervention), hemoglobin (HbA1c – primary outcome variable), blood pressure and weight (secondary outcome) whereas the body mass index (BMI) is a calculated variable. The linear regression analysis will be performed after three months between HbA1c and on the blood glucose results to see the reliability of measurement data and to observe any relationship between the two variables.

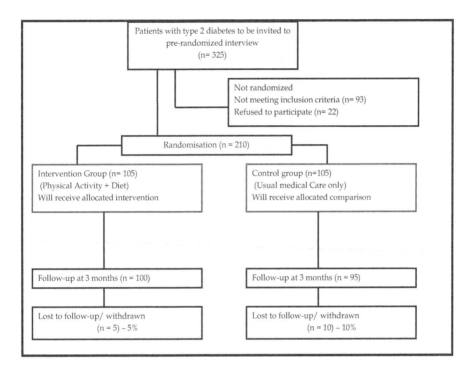

Figure 2. Flow chart describing Randomized Controlled Trial of lifestyle Interventions

Physical activity is a key component of lifestyle modification that can help individuals prevent or control type 2 diabetes. It is considered that diet is probably more important in the initial phases of weight loss, incorporating exercise as part of a weight loss regimen helps maintain weight and prevent weight regain (Klein et al. 2004). In this study, the message will be given to participants to do 30 minutes of moderate physical activity daily (approximately 8000 step count) and it may offer greater benefits to these patients in managing their diabetes (Wright and Royson, 1996).

For measurement of physical activity, the method of step count using pedometer will be used as it has been demonstrated to have a superior validity of step counts over a questionnaire approach in predicting health markers such as BMI and waist circumference (Ewald et al. 2008). The participants will be given pedometer for a week for the measurement of physical activities (step counts). These participants will be instructed to wear the pedometer on a waist belt, either side and wear it from the early morning till they go to bed in the night. The participants will record the start and end time for each day wearing the pedometer and in the evening record the step count showing on the display without resetting the counter. The participants will return a 7-day diary with a record of all the events. Table 2 shows the baseline characteristics of participants in intervention and control group.

Characteristics	Intervention Group (n = 105)	Control Group (n = 105)	P-value
Age (years)	Mean (62.5) ± SD (10.5)	Mean (59.5) ± SD (8.5)	0.78
Sex			
Male	55% (n = 58)	58% (n = 61)	
Female	45% (n = 47)	42% (n = 44)	
Body Mass Index (Kg/m2)	Mean (30.8) ± SD (6.5)	Mean (30.6) ± SD (6.5)	0.40
Physical Activity	95% (8000 steps) 98% (n=103)	-	
Adherence to diet	2% (n = 2)	-	
Baseline Hemoglobin (HbA1c) %	Mean (8.5) ± SD (1.6)	Mean (8.4) ± SD (0)	0.59
Diabetes Medications	Mean (1.75) ± SD (0.8)	Mean (1.82) ± SD (0.8)	0.15

Table 2. Baseline characteristics of intervention and control groups in RCT trial (ref: Medical Record)

12. Method of analysis

12.1. Statistical analysis

The primary outcome will be analysed by an un-paired sample t-test (mean difference between baseline and final HbA1c). The statistical analysis, using STATA will be carried out on an intention to treat basis and that will subject to the availability of data at follow up (after 90 days) as well as at entry level for individual patients. The linear regression analysis will be performed after three months between HbA1c and on the blood glucose results and it is expected that the HbA1c and the self-glucose monitoring via a glucometer will demonstrate a significant relationship ($P < 0.0001$) similar to the findings of Nathan et al. (2008) who reported that the linear regression analysis carried out between the HbA1c and blood glucose (BG) values provided the tightest correlations (BG = $28.7 \times$ A1C – 46.7, $R^2 = 0.84$, $P < 0.0001$), allowing calculation of an estimated average glucose for HbA1C values. The linear regression equations did not differ significantly across subgroups based on age, sex, diabetes type, race/ethnicity, or smoking status.

12.2. Data analysis method

In this study, the thematic analysis of data will be adopted for analysing the data because the method was developed to meet the needs of investigating the experiences, meanings and the reality of the participants (Braun and Clarke, 2006). The method also allows the study to adopt the element from constructionist notions – to investigate the ways in which events, realities, meanings, experiences are the effects of a range of discourses operating within a society. There are five stages to complete this method – it follows the sequence of familiarization, generating initial codes, searching for themes, reviewing themes, defining and naming and preparing the report.

12.3. Sample size estimation

The study sample size was determined based on the assumption of the estimation of Standard Deviation (SD). Therefore, the study design was selected to detect an effect size of 0.5 SD lowering of HbA1c. It was assumed that 10% patients might be lost to follow-up in control group over the period of three months and only 5 % patients will be lost to follow-up in intervention group. This assumption was based on impact of education and advice on lifestyle behavioural modifications to patients and overall popularity of this approach among the diabetic patients in sub-continent to manage their glycemic control.

Taking into consideration all these factors, the following parameters were considered: α = Level of significance test = 0.05, Power = 0.8, m= the follow-up period 90 days (3 months), Standard Deviation (SD) = 0.5, the sample size was calculated for each group to detect an effect size of 0.5 SD. The sample size (N) for each group was =105; therefore, the total, N=210 patients were recruited to participate in both the groups. The figure 2 shows n=210 patients randomized to each group and their progress during double-blinded fenugreek randomized controlled trial.

12.4. Calculation of sample size — An alternate method

Sample Size (N)=$\frac{P1\times(100-P1)+P2\times(100-P2)}{(P1-P2)^2} \times (\alpha,\beta)$

Where,

P1 = % age success expected in intervention group

P2 = % age success on the control group, being different from P1

α = Level of significance test

β = type II error

Assuming that % age success P1 = 95 %, P2 = 90%,

and the factor f (α, β) = f (0.05, 0.5) = 3.8 (source: Table of f (α, β) – EPID6430 course notes)

Sample Size (N)=$\frac{95\times(100-95)+90\times(100-90)}{(95-90)^2}\times(3.8)=209$

13. Clinical settings in pakistan

Diabetic Medical Center, Ayub Medical College, Abbottabad – Pakistan

Patients = patients of type 2 diabetes visiting the medical center

Doctors = doctors working in medical center

14. Minimizing the bias

It is possible that the outcome measures associated with physical activity and diet interventions will be subject to bias particularly when treatment will be in progress or just afterwards. The main difference between usual medical care alone for the patients and usual medical care with physical activity and dietary interventions will occur after 3 months period of trial. In order to reduce the bias, the questionnaire will be sent to patients at home or via e-mail to minimize any chance that their answers might be affected by actual or perceived influence by medical practitioners at clinic.

15. Discussions

The results of this randomized controlled trial will support the research question that lifestyle interventions (physical activity and diet) with usual medical care for type 2 diabetes is more effective than the usual medical care alone. The higher % age of lost to follow up throughout this trial (Figure 2) in those patients with usual medical care (10%) than in those in intervention group (5%) suggests greater satisfaction with physical activity and dietary education and advice. The difference at 3 months follow up is the mean change in HbA1c levels for the intervention group minus the mean change of HbA1c for the control group. Therefore, the positive differences reflect more improvement in those patients following physical activity and dietary guidelines than in those patients with medical care only.

15.1. Testing hypothesis 1 (Primary outcome variable — HbA1c)

The expected changes in HbA1c from baseline values in patients with type 2 diabetes after 3 months will be calculated by unpaired sample t-test. At 3 months follow-up, the patients would show significantly greater improvement and lower values of HbA1c by 1%. This would support the hypothesis 1 that the lifestyle interventions (physical activity and diet) in patients with poorly controlled diabetes will lead to reduction of 1% hemoglobin (HbA1c) in 90 days trial.

These finding are in agreement with the studies by Stratton et al (2000) and the United Kingdom Prospective Diabetes Studies (UKPDS, 1998), suggesting that any reduction in HbA1c is likely to reduce the risk of complications, with the lowest risk being in those with HbA1c values in the normal range (< 6.0%). Therefore, the potential results of this trial which have shown improvement in patients of diabetes by lowering HbA1c by 1% might be expected to provide similar reductions in morbidity.

15.2. Testing Hypothesis 2 (Secondary outcome variable)

The hypothesis 2 will be supported if we can provide evidence that the type 2 diabetic patients after the 90 days trial would reduce 5% weight and consequently the BMI as compared to the these values at baseline. The polynomial regression analysis will be used to generate the reference range models as these models do not make assumptions about linearity of step count with age (Wright and Royson, 1996). It is expected to find a correlation of step count with BMI similar to one of the studies (Ansari, 2009) which provided evidence that relationship between physical activity and BMI was found to be statistically significant in a cross-sectional study of a large sample of population and it was also associated with reduced risk of type 2 diabetes with (RR=0.82; 95% CI=0.68-1.00; P =0.048). The changes in BMI from the base line values will determine the level of reduction in weight and BMI based on physical activity, diet and exercise.

16. Ethical consideration

The scientific validity of the study is a fundamental ethical protection and this study has a scientific merit and clinical value as it aims at using the socio-ecological approach to self-management of type 2 diabetes and will help diabetic patients to control their hemoglobin (HbA1c) and help them to understand the importance of physical activity and healthy diet and to enjoy a healthy lifestyle.

All the patients will be provided clear instruction about the study and informed consent will be obtained and ethical clearance will be taken from a legal authority before conducting this study.

Finally, the main contribution of this trial is to provide health professionals (diabetes care providers) and patients with type 2 diabetes an insight into the ways in which diabetes is viewed and managed in that region of Pakistan which will help them in the self-management and treatment of type 2 diabetes.

17. Conclusion

It has been demonstrated in this study that the level of HbA1c (primary outcome) will reduce by 1% in the patients of poorly controlled type 2 diabetes after the 90 days trial of physical activity and dietary interventions and hence will support the hypothesis and the research question. This study will enhance the relationship between the medical practitioner and the patients of diabetes and will improve the health care system in that region of the country in managing and treating the patients with chronic disease such as diabetes. This study will improve upon the overall functioning of community healthcare clinics to diabetes care in terms of recognizing the symptoms of diabetes to early detection and diagnosis, easy access to community doctors.

Author details

Rashid M. Ansari, John B. Dixon and Colette J. Browning

School of Primary Health Care, Faculty of Medicine, Nursing and Health Sciences, Monash University, Notting Hill, Australia

References

[1] American Diabetes Association ((2000). Clinical practice recommendations 2000. Diabetes Care 23 (Suppl. 1):SS116, 2000., 1.

[2] American Diabetes Association ((2006). Standards of medical care in diabetes. Diabetes Care. 29 (suppl. 1): SS42., 4.

[3] Ansari, R. M. (2009). Effect of physical activity and obesity on type 2 diabetes in middle-aged population. Journal of Environmental and Public Health, , 2009, 4-9.

[4] Beck, A, Scott, J, Williams, P, et al. (1997). A randomized trial of group outpatient visits for chronically older HMO members: the cooperative health care clinic. J Am Geriatr Soc. , 45(5), 543-549.

[5] Blaxter, M. (1990). Health and Lifestyles.London: Tavistock/Routledge.

[6] Brown, S. A. (1990). Studies of educational interventions and outcomes in diabetic adults: A meta-analysis revisited. Patient Education and Counselling, , 16, 189-215.

[7] Brown, S. A, & Hedges, L. V. (1994). Predicting metabolic control in diabetes: a pilot study using meta-analysis to estimate a linear model. Nurs Res , 43, 362-368.

[8] Brownson, R. C, Housemann, R. A, Brown, D. R, et al. (2000). Promoting physical activity in rural communities: walking trail access, use and effects. Am J Pre Med. , 18, 235-241.

[9] Chandler, M. J, Lalonde, C. E, Sokol, B. W, & Hallett, D. (2003). Personal persistence, identity development, and suicide: a study of Native and Non- native North American adolescents. Monogr Soc Res Child Dev.68 (2): vii-viii, , 1-130.

[10] Chin, M. H, Auerbach, S. B, Cook, S, Harrison, J. F, et al. (2000). Quality of diabetes care in community health centers. Am J Public Health , 90, 431-434.

[11] Chin, M. H, Zhang, J. X, Merrell, K, et al. (1998). Diabetes in the African-American Medicare population: morbidity, quality of care, and resource utilization. Diabetes Care , 21, 1090-1095.

[12] Cohen, S, Doyle, W. J, & Skoner, D. P. (1997). Social ties and susceptibility to the common cold. JAMA , 277, 1940-1944.

[13] Davison, C, Smith, G. D, & Frankel, S. (1991). Lay epidemiology and the prevention paradox. Sociol Health Illn , 13, 1-19.

[14] Dignam, J. T, Barrera, M, & West, S. G. (1986). Occupational stress, social support, and burnout among correctional officers. Am. J. COMMUN. Psychol. , 14, 177-193.

[15] Ewing, R, Schmid, T, & Killingsworth, R. (2003). Relationship between urban sprawl and physical activity, obesity, and morbidity. Am J Health Promot. , 18, 47-57.

[16] Fisher, E. B, Brownson, C. A, Tool, O, et al. (2005). Ecological approaches to self-management: The case of diabetes. American Journal of Public Health. , 95, 1523-1535.

[17] Frank, L. D, Engelke, P. O, & Schmid, T. L. (2003). Health and Community Design: The Impact of the Built Environment on Physical Activity. Washington, DC: Island Press.

[18] French, D. P, Senior, V, Weinman, J, et al. (2001). Causal attributions for heart disease: a systematic review. Psychol Health , 16, 77-98.

[19] Frumkin, H, Frank, L, & Jackson, R. (2004). Urban Sprawl and Public Health: Designing, Planning, and Building for Healthy Communities. Washington, DC: Island Press.

[20] Gaede, P, Vedel, P, Larsen, N, Jensen, G. V. H, et al. (2003). Multifactorial intervention and cardiovascular disease in patients with Type 2 diabetes. New England Journal of Medicine, , 348, 383-393.

[21] Glasgow, R. E, Strycker, L. A, Toobert, D, et al. (2000). The Chronic Illness Resources Surveys: A social-ecologic approach to assessing support for disease self-management. Journal of Behavioral Medicine. , 23, 559-583.

[22] Glasgow, R. E, & Eakin, E. G. (1998). Issues in diabetes self-management. In Shumaker, SA et al. (eds). The Handbook of Health Behaviour Change, Springer, New York, , 435-461.

[23] Glasgow, R. E, Toobert, D. J, & Gillette, C. D. (2001). Psychosocial barriers to diabetes self-management and quality of life. Diabetes Spectrum, , 14, 33-41.

[24] Glasgow, R. E, Ruggiero, L, Eakin, E. G, et al. (1997). Quality of life and associated characteristics in a large diverse sample of adults with diabetes. Diabetes Care, , 20, 562-567.

[25] Glasgow, R. E, & Toobert, D. J. (1988). Social environment and regimen adherence among Type II diabetic patients. Diabetes Care, , 11, 377-386.

[26] Glasgow, R. E, Wagner, E, Kaplan, R. M, et al. (1999). If diabetes is a public health problem, why not treat it as one? A population-based approach to chronic illness. Ann. Behav. Med. , 21, 1-13.

[27] Glasgow, R. E. (1995). A practical model of diabetes management and education. Diabetes Care. 18(1), 117-126.

[28] Glasgow, R. E, Orleans, C. T, Wagner, E. H, et al. (2001). Curry SJ, Solberg LI. Does the Chronic Care Model serve also as a template for improving prevention? Milbank Q. , 79(4), 579-612.

[29] Glasgow, R. E, Toobert, D. J, Barrera, M. J, et al. (2005). The Chronic Illness Resources Survey: cross-validation and sensitivity to intervention. Health Educ Res. , 402-409.

[30] Gochman, D. S. (1997). Handbook of Health Behaviour Research II, Plenum Press, NY.

[31] Haire-joshu, D. (1996). Management of Diabetes Mellitus: Perspectives of care across the lifespan. 2nd ed. St. Louis, Mo: C.V. Mosby Co.

[32] Hampson, S. E, Glasgow, R. E, & Strycker, L. (2000). Beliefs versus feelings: a comparison of personal models and depression for predicting multiple outcomes in diabetes. Br J Health Psychol. , 5, 27-40.

[33] House, J. S, Landis, K. R, & Umberson, D. (1988). Social relationships and health. Science , 241, 540-545.

[34] HughnerR.S & Schultz, KS ((2004). Views of Health in the Lay Sector: A Compilation & Review of How Individuals Think about Health. , 8, 395-422.

[35] Huston, S. L, Evenson, K. R, Bors, P, et al. (2003). Neighbourhood environment, access to places for activity, and leisure-time physical activity in a diverse North Carolina population. Am J Health Promot., 18, 58-69.

[36] International Diabetes Federation ((2003). Diabetes prevalence, available online from: http://www.idf.org/home/index.cfm

[37] Jafar, T. H, Chaturvedi, N, & Pappas, G. (2006). Prevalence of overweight and obesity and their association with hypertension and diabetes mellitus in an Indo-Asian population. CMAJ , 175(9), 1071-7.

[38] Johnston, M. E, Gibson, E. S, Terry, C. W, et al. (1984). Effects of labelling on income, work and social function among hypertensive employees. Journal of Chronic Disease, , 37, 417-423.

[39] Kahn, E. B, Ramsey, L. T, Brownson, R. C, et al. (2002). The effectiveness of interventions to increase physical activity: a systematic review. Am J Prev Med. , 22, 73-107.

[40] Kaplan, R. M, Ganiats, T. G, & Sieber, W. J. (1998). The quality of well being scale: Critical similarities and differences with SF-36. International Journal of Quality of Health Care. , 10, 509-520.

[41] Kaplan, R. M, & Toshima, M. T. (1990). The functional effects of social relationships on chronic illness and disability. In Sarason, BS, Sarason, I.G and Pierce, G.R (eds). Social Support: An International View, Wiley, New York, , 427-453.

[42] King, D. K, Glasgow, R. E, Toobert, D. J, et al. (2010). Self-efficacy, problem solving, and social environment support are associated with diabetes self-management behaviours. Diabetes Care , 33, 751-753.

[43] Kirmayer, L. J, Gregory, M, & Tait, L. (2000). The mental health of Aboriginal peoples: transformations of identity and community. Can J Psychiatry. , 45(7), 607-16.

[44] Lorig, K. R, & Holman, H. (2003). Self-management education: history, definition, outcomes, and mechanisms. Ann Behav Med. , 26, 1-7.

[45] Macfarlane, A, & Kelleher, D. (2002). Concepts of illness causation and attitudes to health care among older people in the Republic of Ireland. Soc Sci Med , 54, 1389-400.

[46] Marzilli, G. (1999). The Effects of Social Support on Eating Behaviour in Patients with Diabetes." Available: (http://insulin-pumpers.org/textlib/psyc353.pdf).Retrieved May 25, 2009.

[47] May, P. A, Serna, P, Hurt, L, & Debruyn, L. M. (2005). Outcome evaluation of a public health approach to suicide prevention in an American Indian tribal nation. Am J Public Health., 95(7), 1238-44.

[48] Mckay, H. G, Feil, E. G, Glasgow, R. E, et al. (1998). Feasibility and use of an internet support service for diabetes self-management. Diabetes Educ. , 24, 174-179.

[49] Miller, K. L, & Hirsch, I. B. (1994). Physicians' practices in screening for the development of diabetic nephropathy and the use of glycosy-lated hemoglobin levels. Diabetes Care , 17, 1495-1497.

[50] Narayan, K. M. V. (2005). The Diabetes Pandemic: Looking for the silver lining: Clinical diabetes. , 23, 51-52.

[51] National Health Survey of Pakistan ((1998). Health Profile of the people of Pakistan, Islamabad, Pakistan: Pakistan Medical Research Council., 1990-94.

[52] Norris, S. L, Lau, J, Smith, S. J, et al. (2002). Self-management education for adults with type 2 diabetes: a meta-analysis of the effect on glycemic control. Diabetes Care. , 25, 1159-1171.

[53] Pendleton, D, Schofield, T, & Tate, P. (1984). The Consultation: An Approach to Learning and Teaching. Oxford: Oxford University Press.

[54] Peters, A. L, Legorreta, A. P, Ossorio, R. C, et al. (1996). Quality of outpatient care provided to diabetic patients: a health maintenance organization experience. Diabetes Care, 19, 601-606.

[55] Piette, J. D, Weinberger, M, Kraemer, F. B, et al. (2001). Impact of automated calls with nurse follow-up on diabetes treatment outcomes in a Department of Veterans

Affairs Health care system: a randomized controlled trial. Diabetes Care. , 24, 202-208.

[56] Piette, J. D, Mcphee, S. J, Weinberger, M, et al. (1999). Use of automated telephone disease management calls in an ethnically diverse sample of low-income patients with diabetes. Diabetes Care. , 22, 1302-1309.

[57] Rayappa, P. H. Raju, KNM, Kapur, A et al ((1998). The impact of socio-economic factors on diabetes care. Int J Diab Dev Countries. , 19, 7-15.

[58] Rood, R. P. (1996). Patients and physician responsibility in the treatment of chronic illness: the case of diabetes. American Behavioral Scientist, , 39(6), 729-751.

[59] Roter, D. L, Hall, J. A, Mersica, R, et al. (1998). Effectiveness of interventions to improve patient compliance. Med. Care , 36, 1138-1161.

[60] Sherbourne, C. D, Hays, R. D, & Ordway, L. (1992). Antecedents of adherence to medical recommendations: Results from the medical outcomes study. J. Behav. Med. , 15, 447-468.

[61] Stokols, D. (1996). Translating social ecological theory into guidelines for community health promotion. Am J Health Promot. 10(4), 282-298.

[62] Thompson, S. J, & Gifford, S. M. (2000). Trying to keep a balance: the meaning of health and diabetes in an urban Aboriginal community. Social Science and Medicine, , 51, 1457-1473.

[63] Thompson, O. M, Ballew, C, Resnicow, K, et al. (2004). Food purchased away from home as a predictor of change in BMI z-score among girls. Int J Obes Relat Metab Disord., 28(2), 282-289.

[64] Trento, M, Passera, P, Tomalino, M, et al. (2001). Group visits improve metabolic control in type 2 diabetes: a 2-year follow-up. Diabetes Care. , 24, 995-1000.

[65] Uchino, B. N, Cacioppo, J. T, & Kiecolt-glaser, J. K. (1996). Relationship between social support and physiological processes: A review with emphasis on underlying mechanisms and implications for health. Psychol. Bull. , 119, 488-531.

[66] Wagner, E. H. (1998). Chronic disease management: What will it take to improve care for chronic illness? Effective Clinical Practice. , 1, 1-4.

[67] Wagner, E. H, Austin, B. T, & Von Korff, M. (1996). Organizing care for patients with chronic illness. Milbank Q. , 74, 511-544.

[68] Wagner, E. H, Glasgow, R. E, Davis, C, et al. (2001). Quality improvement in chronic illness care: a collaborative approach. Jt Comm J Qual Improv. 2001; , 27, 63-80.

[69] Weeramanthri, T, Hendy, S, Connors, C, Ashbridge, D, et al. (2003). The Northern Territory Preventable Chronic Disease Strategy- promoting an integrated and life

course approach to chronic disease in Australia. Australian Health Review , 26(3), 31-42.

[70] Wareham, N. J, Byrne, C. D, Williams, R, et al. (1999). Fasting proinsulin concentrations predict the development of type 2 diabetes. Diabetes Care, , 22, 262-270.

[71] Weinberger, M, Kirkman, M. A, Samsa, G. P, et al. (1995). A nurse-coordinated intervention for primary care patients with non-insulin-dependent diabetes mellitus: impact on glycemic control and health-related quality of life. J Gen Intern Med. , 10, 59-66.

[72] WHO Expert Consultation ((2004). Appropriate body-mass index for Asian populations and its implications for policy and intervention. Lancet. , 363, 157-63.

[73] Williams, R, Herman, W, Kinmonth, A. L, et al. (2002). Evidence Base for Diabetes Care. Wiley, Chichester.

[74] Wong, M, Haswell-elkins, M, Tamwoy, E, et al. (2005). Perspectives on clinic attendance, medication and foot-care among people with diabetes in the Torres Strait Islands and Northern Peninsula Area. Australian Journal of Rural Health , 13(5), 172-177.

Chapter 4

Control and Prevention of Obesity and Diabetes Type 2 Through Non-Pharmacological Treatments Based on Marine Products

Daniela Seelenfreund, Pilar Durruty, Nicolas Palou,
Sergio Lobos and Rodrigo González

Additional information is available at the end of the chapter

1. Introduction

Obesity is currently considered as the pandemic of the 21st century and is paradigmatic of non-transmissible chronic diseases, such as type 2 diabetes mellitus (DM2), cardiovascular disease and cancer. Thus, due to its extent, obesity is considered a public health problem that is constantly growing and globally affects both the developed world and developing countries (WHO Prevalence of Diabetes, 2010). In the United States of America (USA) over 30% of the adult population is obese, the numbers in Europe are between 15 and 20 % and in Chile, with a GDP close to $US 20,000 per year, the National Health Survey (Encuesta Nacional de Salud, ENS) of 2010, showed a total prevalence of obesity of 27.4 %, very similar to industrialized countries (ENS, 2010).

All epidemiologic studies show that obesity is greater in subjects with low education and less in individuals with higher education; in Chile, obesity reaches 35% in the former. Additionally, obesity increases with people's age, reaching its highest level in the group of those between 50 – 64 years. However, it is very important to mention the increase in obesity in children and adolescents observed in Europe, in Chile and practically throughout the world, and which is the main cause of the appearance in recent years of a constantly increasing number of type 2 diabetes cases in these age groups (ENS, 2010).

Obesity should be considered as a heterogeneous, multifactorial disease with a genetic base – more than 60 genes involved have been described – however, predisposition to obesity is not higher than 30% and environmental factors of individuals and populations account for 70%. The highest impact factor in the development of obesity is excess food intake and the quality of the diet with high contents of carbohydrates and fats, to which sedentary lifestyles and lack of physical activity are added, both at work and at leisure, a feature common to all populations nowadays.

Among the causes of obesity, mention should be made of aggressive marketing of non-healthy foods, the low price of the so-called "junk food", higher economic income, as well as higher availability of public transportation and of television sets, video games and internet, all of which lead to an increase in sedentary lifestyles at all ages. Obesity *per se* is an independent risk factor for coronary cardiopathy, whereby it has been included by the American Heart Association as a major risk factor. Two important investigations, the Framingham and the Finnish prospective study, confirm the direct association between obesity and coronary mortality.

Visceral obesity is the main causing factor of metabolic syndrome (MS), which has been defined as a group of metabolic risk factors (arterial hypertension, dyslipidemia, glucose intolerance), that are more than randomly interrelated with each other and which directly promote the development of DM2 and cardiovascular disease (CVD). In the USA, health surveys show a sustained increase in the prevalence of MS; thus, the National Health and Nutrition Examination Survey (NHANES) for 1988 – 94 showed a prevalence of 23.1%, while the same survey in 1999 – 2006 reported a worrying increase reaching 34%. The Chilean ENS for 2010 reported very similar figures of 35% (ENS, 2010), while in 2003 it was 22.6%.

Obesity and particularly android or visceral obesity is associated with type 2 diabetes. It should be highlighted that at diagnosis of DM2, 80% of the subjects are obese. While this is true for diabetes in general, it should be considered that 90 – 95% of diabetic patients suffer diabetes type 2 and only 5 to 10% correspond to diabetes type 1, of autoimmune pathogenesis not related to obesity. In our country, only 1% are type 1 diabetic patients.

There is a universal consensus in that obesity is the leading pathogenic factor of pre-diabetes and DM2. Obesity is a determinant of insulin resistance (IR) with compensatory hyperinsulinemia; DM2 becomes manifest when a relative deficiency of insulin secretion is produced.

The International Diabetes Federation estimated a world-wide DM2 prevalence rate of 8.3% for 2011, which will increase to 9.9% by 2030. Some populations, such as Pima Indians from the USA or Mexico and people from the Mauritius Islands with rates higher than 20 – 30% are exceptions. Prevalence is growing explosively, thus the WHO reported that in 2010 there existed 250,000,000 diabetic patients in the world and most remarkably predicted a figure of 333,000,000 for 2025. The same growth is shown in Chilean investigations, with a progressive increase from 5.3% in 1981 to 6.3 in 2003 and 9.4% in 2010. The Chilean survey also shows a clear parallel between prevalence of obesity and DM2 according to age groups (ENS, 2010). The same as with obesity, DM2 is present in higher rates in people with less education and socially more vulnerable groups, which confirms the close association with DM2. It also increases with age, reaching figures close to 20% in elderly subjects.

Mortality for diabetes due to its chronic complications, particularly macrovascular complications and especially coronary death, is among the 10 leading causes of death worldwide, and the seventh cause of death in Chile. Diabetic patients exhibit 8 to 15 time higher frequency of cardiovascular disease (CVD) and 2 to 3 time higher cardiovascular disease mortality than the general population. In the last 40 years, mortality for this cause has decreased in the general population, but not in diabetics. In summary, coronary disease is the main cause of death in DM2 and hyperglycemia is a direct mortality risk factor.

From the above the strong association between obesity, metabolic syndrome and DM2 can be derived, which have common pathogenic mechanisms. It is widely accepted that for prevention of these three pathologies, the main control measures are similar: a healthy diet and increased physical activity.

2. Prevention of DM

It is well known that dietary strategies are needed in order to prevent the onset and control of DM2, at least 80% of the population with DM2 is obese, 75% suffers hypertension and approximately 50% of DM2 patients are dislipidemic (mainly low high-density lipoprotein cholesterol (HDL) and hypertriglyceridemia). General dietary prescriptions for both obese and DM2 patients include well known diets of controlled calorie intake and predominant consumption of certain food groups like vegetables, legumes, fruits and nuts, whole-grain cereals, olive oil, wine and fish.

Risk Prediction Factors for DM2. In 2007, the International Diabetes Federation (IDF) published a consensus on DM2 prevention and defined non-modifiable and modifiable risk factors (Alberti *et al.*, 2007). Among the first are genetic factors, age - at an older age frequency of DM2 is higher - and previous gestational diabetes (about 50% of women with a history of gestational diabetes present DM2 10 years after delivery). Other non-modifiable risk factors are low birth weight children (fetal undernutrition) and big for gestational age babies, who frequently develop obesity as adults and, consequently, diabetes. The main individual modifiable risk factor is obesity, particularly of the android type and, secondly, physical inactivity. There is uncertainty regarding the influence of certain dietary factors, such as a possible involvement of diets that are high in caloric content, saturated fatty acids and low in unsaturated fatty acids and fiber.

Physiopathology of DM2. An important fact for being able to prevent a disease is the existence of a long latency period, which allows the individual to take favorable actions. DM2 meets this requirement, as it has a slow progression and is preceded by identifiable, reversible stages. These begin with an insulin resistance (IR) state with compensatory insulin secretion sufficient to maintain normoglycemia, with hyperinsulinemia values. Subsequently, there begins a progressive fall in insulin levels, when the beta cell is no longer able to maintain hyperfunction, and as insulin secretion deficiency begins, glycemia levels increasingly rise. Initially post-prandial glucose is affected, and later fasting glucose, a state designated as "prediabetes". If no measures are taken, after approximately 10 years of the IR state, clinical DM2 develops. Other physiopathological alterations in DM2 patients that are still under study are the existence of an accelerated gastric emptying and defects in the regulation of feeding, which may explain obesity of these patients.

Search for individuals at risk for DM2. In 2007 international experts established the necessary steps for preventing DM2, based on controlling the modifiable risk factors (Alberti *et al.*, 2007). They defined two groups, separating persons at high risk of developing DM2 from the rest of individuals. Once the former have been identified, it is necessary to measure the risk level with a score, in order to take the necessary actions. For identifying persons over 18 years with a high risk for DM2, a questionnaire is applied which should include the following factors: (android) obesity, age, family history of DM, cardiovascular and in women of gestational diabetes, and the use of diabetogenic drugs (glucocorticoids, adrenergic beta antagonists, thiazides and thyroid hormones). For a precise risk measurement, some models have been proposed, such as the non-invasive, low cost Diabetes Risk Score by Lindström (Lindström & Tuomihleto, 2003), which does not include laboratory tests.

To date, evaluation guidelines recommended by the international organizations to establish with higher certainty a predictive score are still lacking, in order to mathematically select those individuals with higher risk for DM; in the future, this will be a very useful tool. There is no agreement regarding the search mode in children and adolescents, and the risk factors employed are those established for adults: obesity, sedentarism, family history of DM and, additionally, other factors pertaining to adolescents, such as the increase in growth hormone during puberty and presence of polycystic ovary syndrome or hyperandrogenism; in children, low birth weight and growth retardation could be important. A search mode for pregnant women at risk for DM has not been internationally defined either.

The IDF (Alberti *et al.*, 2007) establishes that once persons at risk for DM2 have been identified, the recommendation is to determine fasting and post-load glycemias, which allow detecting cases of glucose intolerance and non-diagnosed DM. In addition, in fasting glycemias ranging between 110-125 mg/dl (impaired fasting glucose, as defined by the IFG), the recommendation is to perform an Oral Glucose Tolerance Test (OGTT) with 75 g glucose. Those persons with glycemia of 140-200 mg/dl are glucose intolerant (GI). Both states are designated as prediabetes and, if no pharmacological and non-pharmacological measures are received, they will develop DM2 in the short term.

2.1. Interventions for preventing or delaying DM2

Prevention with changes in lifestyle. Since the Malmö study, Sweden 1991, there exists evidence demonstrating that changes in lifestyle may delay or prevent DM2, in prediabetic individuals and in those at high risk of developing the disease, even if glycemias are normal. Research carried out in different countries and mainly in Caucasian subjects (the Malmö study, the Finnish Diabetes Prevention Study (DPS) and the US Diabetes Prevention Program (DPP, 2002), achieve similar results, with a decrease in the relative risk (RR) of developing DM2 of 63%, 58% and 58%, respectively (**Table 1**). Studies performed in Chinese individuals, in the city of Da Qing, and in India, Indian Diabetes Prevention Program (IDPP), obtain a smaller risk reduction, of 40% and 29%, respectively. The most remarkable conclusion is that for all studied ethnic groups, it is possible to prevent DM2.

STUDY Country	n	Years of follow-up	Average age (years)	Average BMI (kg/m2)	↓Relative risk of developing DM2
DA QING China	577	6.0	45	25.6	40%
DPS Finland	522	3.2	55	31	58%
DPP USA	3234	2.8	51	34	58%
IDPP India	531	3.0	45.4	25.8	29%

Table 1. Studies on DM2 prevention with lifestyle changes

The five studies discussed have in common that the groups submitted to intervention received feeding advice for reducing weight, plans of structured physical exercise and periodic visits from the medical team for controlling compliance of the indications; on the contrary, the individuals who constituted control groups were only observed, without receiving any special indications. The results of the follow-up of DPS (Lindström *et al.*, 2006) after the end of the three-year intervention period in subjects who had not developed diabetes are very interesting to note, as a 43% reduction of the RR of incidence of DM2 was found. The authors believe that the final success obtained in prediabetic patients is due to the fact that these individuals permanently adopted a healthy lifestyle with greater physical activity, dietary changes and weight loss.

The Da Qing study published similar results to the DPS in an observational study of up to 20 years. It showed a risk reduction of 43% in intolerant patients who were followed for up to 14 years after the end of the 6-year intervention period. The beneficial preventive effect for DM2 does not disappear at the end of the study period, but extends for many more years, probably through permanent lifestyle modifications which were internalized by the individuals.

2.2. DM2 prevention with pharmacological measures

The success obtained in DM2 prevention with changes in lifestyle encouraged many research-ers to perform pharmacological interventions in glucose intolerant patients, especially with pharmacological measures. In Table 2 we summarize findings from several reports on the use of antidiabetic drugs, indicating the number of subjects involved, the years of intervention and the results of these programs on lowering the RR of DM2.

The DPP study (2002) in which glucose intolerant individuals received the metformin but without indications for a change in lifestyle had a much lower efficacy in preventing DM2 (31%), than that obtained with non-pharmacological measures (58%). Very similar achieve-ments were shown by the group with metformin of the IDPP, with the same design and methodology as the previous work. In spite of the relatively modest results with the use of

Study	Drug	n	Years of follow-up	Average age (years)	Average BMI (kg/m2)	↓Relative risk of developing DM2
DPP	Metformin	3234	2.8	51	34	31%
STOP NIDDM	Acarbose	682	3.3	55	31	25%
IDPP	Metformin	531	3.0	46	25.8	26%
ACT NOW	Pioglitazone	602	4.0	52.3	34.3	78%

Table 2. Studies on DM2 prevention with pharmacological interventions

metformin, this insulin-sensitizing medicament is the drug of choice for the pharmacological treatment of the prediabetes state, when additional high-risk factors exist. Presently, it is the drug recommended by the ADA, due to its low side effects and proven therapeutic action.

There are lesser benefits obtained with acarbose in the STOP- NIDDM study with a 25% decrease in RR, in addition to producing marked undesirable digestive side effects and premature drop-out in 31% of the subjects, due to said cause. The use of glitazones is under discussion: Troglitazone and Rosiglitazone have been withdrawn from the market due to cardiovascular risk, and the future of Pioglitazone, used in the ACT NOW study, is uncertain.

Myths or realities in DM2 prevention. Consumption of coffee is widespread throughout the world; it contains caffeine and magnesium which affect glucose metabolism; high coffee intake has been related to lesser risk of DM2 in the USA, Europe and Japan. The phytochemicals in coffee could have a positive effect in slowing down the development of DM2 (van Dam *et al.*, 2006). In Japanese individuals, it was found that consumption of green tea reduces the risk for DM2; flavonoids from vegetables and fruit - also contained in green tea - have insulin activity and increase the action of the hormone (Iso *et al.*, 2006).

One possibility for preventing DM2 would be the administration of vitamins E and C, which improve insulin sensitivity by inhibiting oxidative stress and inflammation, respectively. Rizzo *et al.* (2008), in a controlled study in older men with IFG, found that daily intake of 1000 mg of vitamin E combined with 1000 UI of vitamin C for four weeks, decreased inflammation and improved insulin action, by increasing non-oxidative glucose metabolism, glycemia, insulinemia and lipids. It has been proposed that, due to their potential anti-inflammatory and autoimmune effects, in humans calcium and vitamin D supplements would reduce the incidence of type 1 diabetes and possibly of DM2 (Danescu *et al.*, 2009). The above findings open new prospects for the pharmacological or non-pharmacological prevention of DM2.

DM2 prevention in primary health care. The IDF in its consensus of 2007 (Alberti *et al.*, 2007) addresses this issue and states that "intervention for delaying or preventing diabetes will cause an important reduction of its incidence, its complications and co-morbidities", and recommends controlling the modifiable risk factors:

- - in the whole population and
- - in individuals at high risk of presenting DM2.

For prevention in the population, the IDF suggests to organize National Plans of Diabetes Prevention, adapted to the cultural conditions of each country and supported by existing organized social groups, which might start in nurseries, pre-schools and schools. Programs must have a broad coverage and must be oriented to controlling the two main modifiable risk factors, obesity and sedentarism with the purpose of therapeutic emphasis directed to changes in lifestyle.

3. Dietary strategies for the control of diabetes

The goals of nutritional therapy for diabetes are to prevent and treat complications such as cardiovascular disease, hypertension, nephropathy, obesity and dyslipidemia, and include achieving and maintaining safe or normal blood glucose levels, a normal lipoprotein profile, and an improvement of health through a change of food choices and increased physical activity. A healthy and balanced diet should provide enough calories for daily energy requirements, in order to reduce and/or maintain an acceptable body weight.

3.1. Metabolic control of DM2

It is necessary to know the degree of metabolic control in the type 2 diabetic patient in order to make the proper decisions for his/her treatment (Redsalud, 2006). It has been shown that there is a direct correlation between chronic hyperglycemia and damage to the patient's target systems and organs. The main tests for metabolic control are: glycosylated hemoglobin A1c (HbA1c) and glycemia.

HbA1c. It is currently the best control parameter of glycaemia and reports retrospectively, the glycemia average for a period of 6 to 12 weeks. Two important studies, UKPDS and DCCT, which demonstrated the relationship between metabolic control and appearance or aggravation of microangiopathic complications, employed it as an indicator of the degree of metabolic control. The goal of the treatment is to achieve HbA1c <7%, with individualized variations, the recommendation being that the HbA1c levels should be "the closest to normal, with the least risk of hypoglycemia for the patient". The recommended frequency of check-ups is every 3 months. Considering the heterogeneity of the elderly, goals may be variable, with 7% in a patient in good conditions, to 8.0 - 8.5 % in a patient with limited life expectations due to co-morbidities or with scarce awareness of hypoglycemias.

Glycemia. All patients should be checked with periodic laboratory glycemias or glycemias measured by capillary blood monitors in the clinic. In DM2 patients, this check-up should be carried out every three months. The goals or targets required for pre-prandial and post-prandial glycemias appear in **Table 3.** Capillary glycemias assessed by the patient through self-monitoring are necessary only in DM2 patients on insulin treatment; the usefulness of self-monitoring has not been demonstrated in DM2 patients with oral treatment.

Glycosylated hemoglobin A1c	< 7 %
Pre-prandial glycemias	70 - 130 mg/dl
Post-prandial glycemias	160 - 180 mg/dl

Table 3. Metabolic Goals

Target organ compromise

Retina. The fundus study should be performed at diagnosis of DM2. If normal, it should be repeated annually; if altered, the patient should be referred to a specialist.

Renal compromise. Assessment of plasma creatinine and calculation of glomerular filtration should be performed at diagnosis of DM2 and, if normal, should be repeated annually. Determination of proteinuria is performed at diagnosis of DM2; if negative, a microalbuminuria test is requested. Urinary albumin excretion (UAE) is quantified with the albumin/creatinine ratio in a random urine sample. UAE values between 30 and 300 mg/g should be repeated; microalbuminuria is diagnosed when 2 out of 3 samples continue to be altered. If the UAE values are <30 mg/g, the check-up can be performed annually.

Neuropathy and arteriosclerosis of the lower limbs. The clinical examination is conducted with exploration of feet and testing of tactile and vibratory sensitivity, reflexes and peripheral pulses. This examination is conducted at the patient's diagnosis; if no alterations exist, it should be systematically repeated once a year. In this examination, it is advisable to include the orthostatism test.

Detection and prevention of cardiovascular disease (CVD). DM in general is a risk factor for CVD and DM2 is associated with other factors which form part of the pre-diabetic status and which exert negative interrelations leading to a more precocious and severe CVD. Detection and control of these factors forms part of the treatment of DM; the most important are arterial hypertension and dyslipidemia.

Arterial hypertension. Diabetic patients have a high risk of CVD starting from the pre-hypertension stage, which also contributes to microvascular damage. Its optimized treatment reduces micro- and macrovascular complications of DM. It is essential to guarantee detection, control and treatment of hypertension. The goals to be achieved are < 130/ 80 mm Hg and, in nephropaths, < 125/75 mm Hg.

Dyslipidemia. Lipid alterations are a known risk factor for CVD and are more aterogenic in DM. The most important goal is to correct LDL cholesterol. Added to this is the so-called "aterogenic" dyslipidemia of the diabetic and pre-diabetic patient: elevated triglycerides, low HDL cholesterol and small, dense particles of LDL cholesterol. This explains why detection and treatment of lipid alterations is a main part of the check-up and follow-up of DM2. Lipid profiles should be included in the initial evaluation of DM2. If the result is normal, it should be repeated once a year. The goals to be achieved are: triglycerides <150 mg/dl, HDL >40 mg/dl in men, >50 in women and LDL <100 in primary CVD prevention and <70 in secondary CVD prevention.

With the aim of achieving an optimal metabolic control and prevention of micro- and macro-angiopathic complications, all patients should be encouraged to adhere to a healthy diet, low in cholesterol and saturated fatty acids and high in dietary fiber. Additionally, regular physical activity for 150 minutes per week, fractionated in 5 days, should be promoted.

3.2. Nutritional plan for DM2

Programmed diet (ADA, 2004) is one of the pillars of the treatment of DM2; without it, a proper metabolic control is not achieved, and the patient should permanently adhere to it. In some cases, together with exercise for some time, they both constitute sufficient total treatment for the disease.

Nutritional requirements. Nutritional requirements of persons with diabetes are similar to those of individuals without the disease. Calculation of total calories depends on the physical activity and the nutritional status of the patient. For an estimation of daily calories, the factors listed in **Table 4** are used.

In overweight or obese individuals, a weight loss of 5-10% of the present weight improves blood pressure and glycemic and lipid levels. Knowing the composition of the foods, the ingredients of kitchen recipes and the amounts that should be eaten, it is possible to design the dietary plan and apply the diet for the family group.

Nutritional status	Physical activity		
	Sedentary	Moderate	Intense
Obese (BMI >30 kg/m²)	20-25	30	35
Overweight (BMI >25-29.9 kg/m²)	26-29	28	30
Normal (BMI 20-24-9 kg/m²)	30	35	40
Lean (BMI<20 kg/m²)	35	40	45-50

Table 4. Caloric recommendations for adults. Calories/ kg of acceptable body weight

Carbohydrates (CH). The percentage of carbohydrate calories varies, it is individual and based on eating habits, targeted glycemia and lipids. The recommended range is between 55% and 60% of the total daily calories. Restriction of carbohydrates to less than 130 grams/day is not recommended, since the brain and the nervous system have an absolute requirement for glucose as a source of energy. In the dietary plan, it is advisable to leave out simple sugars (honey, panela, molasses, sugar) or lower them in well-controlled patients to <5 g per day.

Lipids. In the type 2 diabetic patient, elevations in very low density lipoprotein (VLDL) concentrations, reductions in high density lipoprotein (HDL) concentrations and elevations in the low density fraction (LDL) may be found. Type 2 diabetics may have an altered lipid profile, notwithstanding a good glycemic control.

The main goal in lipid intake is to reduce consumption of saturated fatty acids and trans fatty acids. Lipids should account for less than 30% of the total daily caloric intake. Foods containing monounsaturated and polyunsaturated fatty acids should be preferred in order to comply with the recommendations. Less than 7% of the calories provided by saturated (SFA) and *trans* fatty acids is recommended. SFAs are the main source of formation of LDL cholesterol and are found in fatty meats, dairy products and eggs. *Trans* fatty acids are produced by hydrogenating vegetable or fish oils in order to achieve a more solid texture.

Monounsaturated fatty acids (MFA) are recommended in a proportion of 13%, especially in the *cis* configuration, as found in olive oil, sesame, nuts and peanuts. MFAs may be beneficial in the control of blood lipids and of cardiovascular diseases. It is indicated that less than 10 % of the calories should be provided by polyunsaturated fatty acids (PFA), which are found in vegetable oils such as corn, sunflower, safflower and soybean oils. Omega 3 eicosapentenoic and docosahexenoic fatty acids (EPA and DHA) present in fish have a beneficial effect on triglycerides. It is recommended not to exceed an intake of 200 mg of cholesterol per day. Consumption of fish or fish oil containing omega-3 polyunsaturated fatty acids (PUFAs) reduce the risk of coronary heart disease, decrease mild hypertension, prevent certain cardiac arrhythmia and lower the incidence of diabetes. Omega-3 PUFAs play a vital role in the development and function of the nervous system and photoreception. Dietary lipids should be lowered if weight loss is desired; if this dietary scheme is maintained for a long term, it contributes to weight loss and to ameliorate dyslipidemia.

The recommended lipid composition in the diet of a type 2 diabetic patient is set forth in **Table 5.**

< 7% of the calories: saturated (SFA) and trans fatty acids
<10% of the calories: polyunsaturated fatty acids (PFA)
13% of the calories: monounsaturated fatty acids (MFA)
Omega 3 fatty acids (cis configuration) 0.15 g/day

Table 5. Contribution of dietary fatty acids in a DM2 patient

Proteins. Proteins should account for 15-20 % of total caloric intake, 0.8 – 1.0 g/Kg of body weight; dietary protein intake must be balanced and rich in essential amino acids. According to the dietary guidelines, the intake of protein in the usual range does not appear to be associated with the development of diabetic nephropathy, although it is advisable to avoid intakes over 20 % of the total daily energy.

The Recommended Dietary Allowance (RDA) indications for the general population of 0.8 g of proteins of high biological value, per kg of weight per day in the adult, are still followed. Proteins of high biological value provide all of the essential amino acids and in the amounts required by the body; they are the proteins of animal origin, all types of meat (beef, pork, fish, etc), milk and eggs. When the drop in glomerular filtration is initiated, proteins should not be restricted beyond 0.6 g/kg/day in order not to cause malnutrition. In the highly uncompensated type 2 diabetic patient, there could occasionally be a loss of body proteins.

Glycemic index. It is established as the incremental area under the glycemia curve produced by the intake of a standard amount of available CHs of a food (usually 50 g), in relation to the same amount of carbohydrates from a standard source (glucose or white bread). Recommendation is to prefer foods with low glycemic index (legumes, green vegetables).

Dietary fiber. Soluble fiber of vegetables, legumes and fruit (pectin) helps to control not only glycemia but also lipids, and should be accompanied by an increase in water intake. Fibers also help satiety. Processed foods tend to decrease the amount of available fiber. Complex carbohydrates, which also have a high percentage of soluble dietary fiber, are present in legumes, vegetables and fruits, and should be included in a healthy diet.

Sweeteners. Non-caloric sweeteners such as saccharin, aspartame, acesulfame K, sucralose, estevioside are accepted as safe, as long as their accepted daily intake is observed.

Sodium. Individuals differ in sensitivity to sodium intake, related to arterial pressure. Sodium recommendation is the same as for the general population: not more than 2.4 g/day, equivalent to 6.0 g/day of NaCl.

Alcohol. The same recommendations as for the general population are valid. Never to drink on an empty stomach and to prefer red wine due to its phenol (antioxidant) content; the maximal recommended portion is not more than 2 cups per day in men and not more than one in women. 100 ml of wine contain 9-13 g of alcohol, and one gram of alcohol provides 7 calories. Alcohol abstention is recommended during pregnancy, in hypertriglyceridemia, pancreatitis, arterial hypertension or neuropathy. If the individual with diabetes is abstemious, he/she will be advised not to initiate this practice. Fruit and vegetable intake provides a suitable amount of antioxidants.

Vitamins and Minerals. A suitable dietary intake provides vitamins and minerals in sufficient amounts and no supplementation is necessary. However, there are some exceptions: individuals on chronic hypocaloric diets, which should be supplemented with iron and B-Complex vitamins; iron, folate and calcium supplements are recommended to pregnant women; calcium supplement is recommended to women with osteoporosis; and undernourished subjects are advised to take supplements appropriate to the deficiency they present. Vitamin supplementation with antioxidants (vitamins E, C and A) is not advisable as a routine, due to lack of evidence and safety and long-term safety. Chromium, Selenium, Zinc and Manganese are contained in the usual diet, while supplements are recommended only when patients have a deficiency.

The nutritional plan detailed for DM2 is also recommended for individuals who are obese, insulin-resistant, pre-diabetic and carriers of metabolic syndrome, in order to prevent them from developing DM2.

To summarize, one of the key measures to achieve control targets in patients with diabetes is a diet plan, as there is ample evidence that the goals are not achieved if patients fail non-pharmacologic measures, diet and physical activity.

4. Nutrition and social behavior

The drastic and long-term changes in eating habits that are needed in order to prevent and control these diseases require a highly motivated and educated population with the economic means and a strong personal commitment to follow and maintain these indications. Changing dietary habits may be a very difficult task to accomplish and constant support is needed from health professionals who should develop individual therapeutic programs for each patient according to their personal lifestyle requirements, tastes or cultural backgrounds.

Why is it so difficult to achieve this change to healthy eating habits? In the first place it is important to understand that eating is not an isolated behavior, as in all societies it is part of the cultural context that defines what is considered edible or appropriate (or not) for each member of any particular group. Contreras & Grace (2005) suggest the presence of a food culture that accompanies any food system, which is defined as follows: "the set of representations, beliefs, knowledge and practices inherited and / or learned that are associated to food and that are shared by individuals of a given culture or a social group within a culture". In addition to keeping alive and avoiding overt hunger, food all over the world and in all possible settings is also used to keep and classify human relationships, indicate social status, enhance political, business and economic relations, provide praise and punishment, prevent and treat physical and mental disease, to indicate religious adherence or membership, to evidence emotions and even morals. As illustrated above, the underlying development of attitudes, from infancy to old age, in pregnancy and disease, for adolescents and adults influence food behavior and are determined by culture, economics, food technology, politics, the family and recently, by mass media. Consequently, to achieve significant impact, education in nutrition and dietetics also requires knowledge of the socio-cultural aspects of eating as well as its basic scientific aspects, and the professional providing nutrition services and education in the community needs an understanding of these facts (Bass *et al.*, 1979). Briefly, food and food consumption patterns underlie the social fabric in all societies and hence its cultural importance cannot be underestimated.

Second, the social act of eating has changed along the millennia of humankind; therefore it is of use to put the nutritional transitions into a historical context. From a long history of omnivorism of hunter-gatherers (mainly plants supplemented with occasional meat), that shaped our physiology to the present day, humans have moved through several important transitions in their nutrition. Omnivorism probably required cooperation between members of a species that is rather ill-equipped compared to other predators, possibly setting the stage for social patterns for providing and distributing food (Aguirre, 2010). These conditions selected among our ancestors those individuals endowed with genes that permitted the accumulation of calories in times of surplus, and survive in times of low access to food or starvation (Aguirre, 2010).

Later, approximately 15.000 to 10.000 B.P. a major nutritional transition occurs as an adaptation to the higher temperatures of the postglacial era (and the associated decrease of large prey for hunting) which leads to the development of agriculture (Smith & Munro, 2009). The introduction of staple food lead to the establishment of villages and an increase of the human population and a shift to meals based on cereals (i.e. carbohydrates) and a decrease of protein intake. As a result, on a global scale humans on average became approximately 20 cm shorter with a decreased life expectancy due to chronic malnutrition of micronutrients. Also, specific diseases related to agricultural labor and food processing appeared, such as arthritis, skeleton deformities and dental abrasion, particularly in women (Aguirre, 2010). The establishment of sedentary societies also set the stage for classes with differential foods, creating small well-fed upper classes with large, fat bodies and a majority of the population with the short and lean phenotype of poverty, fed a low variety of (or a single) cereal or tuber staple (Aguirre, 2010).

The next nutritional transition comes about with the industrial revolution, which initially causes a severe drop in the quality of life for the large majority of the population in the western world. The new technologies completely change the methods of producing, distributing and consuming foods. The modern relocation of edible plants throughout the world introduces the concept of plantations, and worldwide distribution of some edible products such as sugar, coffee, tea and potatoes, among others (Aguirre, 2010). The economic powers involved provoke colonial wars, and in the long run, create the industrial food production with large scale food transportation and storage, a panoply of additives (flavorings or dyes) and stabilizers, and the disappearance of seasonality of fruits and vegetables and local food production, that charac- terizes the modern food production of in our days.

The genetic makeup of our species has not changed at the pace of these nutritional transitions, so we are now faced with a large population, living in a largely industrial-urban setting that still maintains those biological features that constituted an advantage for survival in the past. Although there are 870 millions of people suffering hunger today (http://faostat3.fao.org/home/index.html), for the first time in human history, a large segment of the population has access to a large supply of calories in the form of carbohydrates and fats, albeit, not to a healthy diet with low fat proteins and micronutrients. Finally, this nutritional transition has happened so fast that the shift from undernourishment to obesity has occurred within just two genera- tions. Indeed, in developing countries, it is not uncommon that an individual, who experienced undernourishment during childhood, is today an obese adult with overweight children. Therefore, in a completely different context, our genetic makeup in an era of surplus calories and changing lifestyles provides the basis for the worldwide epidemic of obesity and diabetes.

As pointed out at the beginning of this section, a highly motivated and educated popula- tion with the economic means and a strong personal commitment to follow and maintain the indications is needed to revert this situation. Low levels of education of mothers also tend to result in children that spent more time watching TV and eat a higher amount of fat and calorie-rich snacks and "junk food", highlighting the importance of enhancing school-based and community-based actions to promote healthy eating and physical activi- ty addressed to children and young people (Aranceta et al., 2003). Also, in the face of in- creasing food prices, many people with lower incomes do not have a realistic possibility of choosing an appropriate diet.

Since the general population in most developing countries such as Chile, is not able to keep these recommendations in the long term for any of the above reasons, several kinds of dietary interventions have been proposed. These include low calorie foods and foods containing high-quality ingredients such as peptides derived from fish. Some of these strategies include the replacement of red meat and its derivatives by fish and white meat, the reduction of the total fat intake (saturated fat) and replacement by the use of other oils (such as olive oil) and a higher intake of dietary fiber, replacing white bread with whole grain bread. Here we propose to include marine-derived proteins, specifically fish-derived protein hydrolysates as high biological value proteins of low cost as dietary supplements or ingredients, as a means of preventing obesity and diabetes.

5. Marine-derived protein

5.1. General aspects

Seafood and fish are sources of high biological value proteins, unsaturated essential fatty acids, vitamins and antioxidants, minerals or trace metals and physiological beneficial amino acids and peptides. Additional components in seafood may be of importance for the development of life style diseases like coronary heart disease. There is ample literature on marine-derived peptides (salmon and other fish) with biological activity against obesity, DM2 and cardiovas-cular disease, which leads to the proposal of using protein concentrates produced by enzymatic hydrolysis from co-products of the fish industry that may contain these peptides. Several research groups, including ourselves, are concentrated on generating an application or nutraceutical biological functionality of these products.

Different strategies have been studied for recovering protein from the marine products industry, as for example fish protein hydrolysates (FPHs, by its acronym in English). These treatments are obtained by solubilizing the raw protein, *via* peptide bond breaks which release smaller peptides and free amino acids, that can then be separated and re-covered. In this type of application protein recovery by enzymatic hydrolysis is chosen, because this treatment gives rise to a final product of higher digestibility than untreated protein (Aurrekoetxea & Perera, 2002).

Several studies reveal that proteins derived from hydrolysis of marine products are of high nutritional value, rich in essential amino acids and even similar to proteins from beef (Kristinsson & Rasco, 2000). It has also been observed that hydrolysates, treated with commercial enzymes, exhibit functional characteristics (solubility, fat absorption, water absorption and stability of the emulsion) consistent with potential uses as emulsifying agents, and absorbing agents, being potentially competitive with existing protein hydroly-sates, such as dairy products and vegetables, which are currently available on the market (Sathivel *et al.*, 2005).

Enzymatic digestion of proteins of marine origin results in FPH. Among the problems of obtaining the FPH, is the extreme susceptibility to oxidation of fats, and the presence of these oil residues which generate unpleasant odors and flavors from an organoleptic viewpoint (Hoyle & Merritt, 1994).

Protein hydrolysates also have non-food applications such as power supply for the growth of microorganisms such as yeast hydrolysates or casein. They can also be used eventually as plant fertilizers and also used in cosmetics for hair treatment (due to its suggested effect of strengthening of hair) (Vioque & Millan, 2005).

Enzymatic hydrolysis has clear advantages over traditional acid or alkaline chemical hydrolysis, for the following reasons (Guadix *et al.*, 2000):

- Selectivity. Enzymes are specific for a particular type of chemical bond, and the appearance of degradation products is not common. In contrast, the low selectivity of the acidic and basic treatments inevitably leads to the appearance of degradation products that are difficult to control and may be toxic.

- Moderate temperature and pH conditions. Enzymatic hydrolysis generally proceeds in the range of 40 to 60°C and pH of 4.0 to 8.0.

- No foreign substances are added. Chemical hydrolysis processes are carried out with strong acids or bases, which are then neutralized, thereby significantly raising the salt content of the product.

- Maintain the nutritional value. There is no degradation of the components, while alkaline hydrolysis destroys the amino acids arginine and cysteine, and acid hydrolysis removes tryptophan and deaminates serine and threonine.

As a result of biological hydrolysis, high-protein, low-fat FPHs can be obtained, which are completely soluble products (Aurrekoetxea & Perera, 2002).

5.2. Physiological effects of marine-derived peptides and aminoacids

Potent peptides with high anti-hypertensive activities (inhibitors of angiotensin I-converting enzyme or ACE) and peptides which may modulate central neuropeptide levels have been isolated from fish hydrolysates (Yoshikawa *et al.*, 2000; Sorensen *et al.*, 2004). Marine low molecular weight components antioxidants (tocopherols, CoQ10, selenium, taurine) have attracted special attention due to their possible prevention of low-density lipoprotein (LDL) oxidation. Fish proteins have also been shown to inhibit LDL oxidation in rat models (Kondo *et al.*, 2000).

It has been documented that peptides obtained from fish muscle digests possess potent inhibitory activity against ACE and antihypertensive properties (Galardy *et al.*, 1984; Kohama *et al.*, 1996). For assessment of relative antihypertensive activities of two peptides (LKPNM and LKP) derived from bonito fish to that of captopril, administered orally to SHR rats to monitor time-course changes of blood pressures (Fujita & Yoshikawa, 1999). Both LKPNM and captopril showed maximal decrease of blood pressure 4 h after oral administration and their efficacies lasted until 6 h post-administration. In sharp contrast, however, maximal reduction of blood pressure occurred as early as 2 h after administration of LKP. When compared on molar basis, antihypertensive activities of LKPNM and LKP accounted for 66% and 91% relative to that of captopril, respectively, whereas *in vitro* ACE-inhibitory activities of LKPNM and LKP were very low compared with that of captopril. It is of interest to note that both of these peptides exerted remarkably higher antihypertensive activities *in vivo* despite weaker *in vitro* ACE-inhibitory effects, using captopril as the reference drug (Fujita & Yoshikawa, 1999). Such peptides may be regarded as healthy components (through endogenous metabolism) of fish muscles and additionally may be produced as ingredients or diet supplements.

Amino acids (taurine) and peptides (ACE -inhibitors) are beneficial components from seafood and hence components in possible ingredients in functional foods. Seafood contains high levels of the amino acid taurine and the consumption of seafood has been shown to increase its serum concentration (Laidlaw *et al.*, 1990; Kim *et al.*, 1996). The suggestion of a possible association between fish intake and reduced cardiovascular risk through the beneficial effects of proteins and taurine, in addition to omega n-3 fatty acids, has been put forward (Mizushima *et al.*, 1997; Yamori *et al.*, 1994).

In humans, taurine is regarded to be a conditionally essential amino acid, as its physiological concentration can be partly regulated endogenously. Taurine is known to have several positive effects on the cardiovascular system, as described in a broad review by Niittynen *et al.* (1999). Firstly, taurine has antioxidant activity. This may reduce the production of proinflammatory products. Secondly, taurine has been shown to lower blood pressure in borderline hypertensive patients. It has also been reported that taurine can improve cardiac performance, reduce blood cholesterol values and suppress platelet aggregation (Niittynen *et al.*, 1999). A protective role from both taurine and ACE inhibitors has been found in age-related progressive renal sclerosis in 24 and 30 months old rats. Taking into account the antioxidant properties of taurine, these data suggest a role for ROS in age-related progressive renal fibrosis, perhaps through interactions with de TGF-β1 pathway (Iglesias-de la Cruz *et al.*, 2000). Although commonly used as a dietary supplement in the Far East, the potential advantages of dietary taurine consumption /supplementation have not been recognized in the Western World (Stapleton *et al.*, 1998).

Frozen-preserved commercial diets have been shown to maintain plasma taurine concentration, whereas the heat-processed diets do not (Kim *et al.*, 1996; Dragnes *et al.*, 2009). On the other hand, a significant correlation was found between the results of the biological assessment of the nutritional value of processed protein and of taurine content in the liver and urine of rats (Lipka *et al.*, 1993).

5.3. Improvement of FPHs through the use of enzymes

The functional properties of FPHs can be improved by the use of specific enzymes and by the choice of the hydrolysis conditions, such as time, temperature and pH. In this way partial hydrolysis can be achieved. There are a number of different commercial proteolytic enzymes that can be used to produce hydrolysates (Liceaga-Gesualdo & Li-Chan, 1999).

The addition of exogenous enzymes to the hydrolytic process makes it more controllable and reproducible. Consequently, different commercial proteolytic enzymes have been tested on a variety of marine substrates. The preferred commercial enzymes are proteases of bacterial origin, such as Alcalase, Neutrase, Protamex (bacterial proteases trade names), but also the plant proteases such as papain (commercially called Corolase L-10), present good yields in hydrolytic processes (Aspmo, 2005).

All enzymes used for hydrolyzing proteins of marine origin have to be of food grade, and if they are of bacterial origin, the production organism needs to be non-pathogenic. The choice of enzyme is usually determined by a combination of effectiveness and economy (Kristinsson & Rasco, 2000). Major factors in the choice of enzymes are the organoleptic and functional characteristics of the final food product.

5.4. Organoleptic properties of the hydrolysate

Although enzymatic hydrolysis of marine proteins produces peptides with desirable functional properties, it has the disadvantage of generating bitterness. This is a common problem with FPHs, and is the main reason for its low acceptance as a food ingredient. The mechanism for the development of bitterness is not yet clear, but it is widely accepted that the hydrophobic amino acids of the peptides are the main factor. The hydrolysis of proteins results in the exposure of internal hydrophobic peptides which are able to interact rapidly with the taste buds, resulting in the detection of bitter taste. However, extensive hydrolysis to produce free amino acids reduces the bitterness of peptides, because hydrophobic peptides are much bitterer compared with a blend of free amino acids, which are though, undesirable from a functional point of view. A strict control of the degree of hydrolysis in any experimental system is therefore desirable to prevent the development of bitter taste and also for the retention of functional properties (Kristinsson & Rasco, 2000; Liaset *et al.*, 2003; Benitez *et al.*, 2008).

Proteases have different specificity for the amino acids they cut, so the choice of the most appropriate enzyme or mixture of enzymes depends on the raw material subjected to hydrolysis, and may affect the degree of bitterness. For instance, enzymes with a high preference for hydrophobic amino acids, such as Alcalase, are often preferred and may yield products with low bitterness. The use of exopeptidases, instead of endoproteases, may also be useful in reducing the bitterness of the FPH, particularly if exopeptidases separating hydrophobic amino acids from bitter peptides are used. However, for an enzyme preparation to be effective in protein hydrolysis, both exopeptidases and endopeptidases are required. Many studies have shown that preparations containing proteolytic exopeptidases and endopeptidases produce less bitter peptides than single proteases. The addition of exopeptidases to the process often eliminates the bitter taste of the hydrolysates (FitzGerald & O`Cuinn, 2006).

The ideal method for the quantification of the bitterness of a hydrolysate is the use of a sensory evaluation panel. This is a time-consuming activity and requires an appropriate number of panelists trained to detect such bitterness, in order to obtain statistically relevant data (Fitz-Gerald & O`Cuinn, 2006; Seo *et al.*, 2008).

5.5. Use of antioxidants in the hydrolysis

Oils and fatty products generally undergo oxidation during production and storage. A major problem of the preparation of FPHs is their extreme susceptibility to such oxidation fats (Hoyle & Merritt, 1994). This oxidation process in food causes a sequence of unfavorable changes, consisting mainly in deterioration of the sensory properties of the product such as rancidity, changes in color and texture and reduced nutritional value. It also increases health risks, along with economic losses and may even influence the development of bitter flavors (Palić & Lucan, 1995; Valenzuela et al., 2003; Gramza & Korczak, 2005; Mendis et al., 2005; Dong et al., 2008).

Marine oils are rich in polyunsaturated fatty acids (PUFAs), especially of the ω3 family such as EPA and DHA, however diets containing these oils are more susceptible to oxidation than those containing other types of oils, because of their high concentrations of long chain PUFAs; the aforementioned examples are DHA and EPA (Gonzalez et al., 1992; Fritsche & Johnston, 1988; Wanasundara & Shahidi, 1998).

PUFA degradation *via* chain reaction mechanisms of free radicals, results in changes of smell and taste (rancidity) of edible oils and oil-containing foods. The chemical reactions involved in oxidative processes require low activation energy, and do not significantly change their ranges at low storage temperatures; therefore, it is necessary to delay the onset of oxidation of the marine oil to maintain its flavor and odor (Wanasundara & Shahidi, 1998; Ahn et al., 2007).

5.6. Antioxidants

Antioxidants, natural and synthetic, are commonly used by the food processing industry, to prolong the storage stability of food. The main commonly used synthetic antioxidants are butylhydroxybutilanisol, butylated hydroxytoluene, propyl gallate and tertiary butylhydro-quinone (BHA, BHT, PG and TBHQ, respectively, for their acronyms in English). Natural antioxidants such as tocopherols, rosemary extracts (Herbalox, commercial product) and ascorbic acid are often preferred (Gramza & Korczak, 2005; Yu et al., 2006).

5.7. Preliminary trials

Preliminary tests of the organoleptic properties of enzymatic hydrolysis of marine proteins with different commercial enzymes, among them Alcalase, and Colorasa Protamex (papain) and different commercial antioxidants, showed greater acceptability of the process than with the protease Colorasa L-10. These results were observed after organoleptic analysis of the obtained products in trials with healthy volunteers (unpublished results).

While the use of antioxidants improves the stability of the oil fraction obtained together with the protein fraction, products derived from an antioxidant-free process were more acceptable (organoleptic properties) than those obtained in a process in which antioxidants were are used, although the oil fraction underwent faster oxidation (unpublished results). These results suggest that the addition of antioxidants is not of vital importance in the course of an organo-leptically suitable product with a high proportion of proteins of marine origin.

6. Concluding comments

In this chapter we present general data concerning the worldwide epidemic of obesity and diabetes and discuss the present day goals of metabolic control of affected patients. The current strategies used for prevention of the development of prediabetes and diabetes are discussed and a brief up-to-date review of summarizes the dietary strategies for the nutrition of diabetic patients.

In the following section we briefly describe the main impact of historic nutritional transitions and illustrate how the social impact of present day food production, distribution and consumption is exacting a high toll on public health (and also on the environment). To amend this general pattern, large changes of society on a global scale are needed. Since these do not seem realistic in the short term, alternative strategies to address particular problems are suggested, such as nutritional intervention with high quality nutrients of low economic value such as supplementing foods with marine-derived protein hydrolysates.

A discussion of the different procedures for obtaining fish derived protein hydrolysates is presented, centered on the advantages of enzymatic hydrolysis, with respect to chemical procedures. The use of antioxidants during the hydrolysis process is also analyzed and not found to be essential for obtaining a high quality product. The organoleptic properties of hydrolysates obtained by our group have proven acceptable in trials to healthy volunteers. In addition, fish derived protein hydrolysates may contain peptides and/or aminoacids which may bear additional beneficial effect.

To summarize, healthy dietary habits are part of the necessary lifestyle to prevent obesity and DM2; an increased intake of marine products is also recommended as a means to control risk factors of cardiovascular disease of DM2 patients.

Author details

Daniela Seelenfreund[1*], Pilar Durruty[2], Nicolas Palou[1], Sergio Lobos[1] and Rodrigo González[1]

1 Department of Biochemistry, Faculty of Chemical and Pharmaceutical Sciences, University of Chile, Providencia, Santiago, Chile

2 Diabetes Unit, Department of Medicine, Faculty of Medicine, University of Chile, Santiago, Chile

References

[1] Aguirre, P. (2010). Ricos flacos y gordos pobres: la alimentación en crisis. 1rst Ed. Capital Intelectual S.A., Buenos Aires, Argentina.

[2] Ahn, J, Grün, I, & Mustapha, A. (2007). Effects of plant extracts on microbial growth, color change, and lipid oxidation in cooked beef. Food Microbiol, , 24, 7-14.

[3] Alberti KGMZimmet P, Shaw J, (2007). International Diabetes Federation: a consensus on Type 2 diabetes prevention. Diabetic Medicine, , 24, 451-463.

[4] American Diabetes Association(2004). Nutrition Principles and Recommendations in Diabetes.. oi: 10.2337/diacare.27.2007.S36 Diabetes Care January 2004 no. suppl 1 s36., 27

[5] Aranceta, J, Pérez-rodrigo, C, & Ribas, L. Serra-Majem, Ll, (2003). Sociodemographic and lifestyle determinants of food patterns in Spanish children and adolescents: the enKid study. Eur J Clin Nutr, 57: Suppl 1, SS44., 40.

[6] Aspmo, S. (2005). Enzymatic hydrolysis of Atlantic cod (Gadusmorhua L.) viscera. Process Biochem, , 40, 1957-1966.

[7] Aurrekoetxea, G, & Pereira, M. (2002). Aprovechamiento de recursos pesqueros infrautilizados para la obtención de alimentos mejorados para el cultivo de peces. Boletín del Instituto Español de Oceanografía, , 18, 87-93.

[8] Bass, M. A, Wakefield, L, & Kolasa, K. (1979). Community nutrition and individual food behavior. Publisher Burgess Pub. Co., Minneapolis (USA).

[9] Benítez, R, Ibarz, A, & Pagan, J. (2008). Hidrolizados de proteína: procesos y aplicaciones. Acta Bioquímica Clínica Latinoamérica, , 42, 227-237.

[10] Contreras, J, & Gracia, M. (2005). Alimentación y Cultura: perspectivas antropológicas. Editorial Ariel. Barcelona, Spain. (Ibid. 2005: 96).

[11] Danescu, L. G, Levy, S, & Levy, J. and diabetes mellitus. Endocrine, , 35, 11-17.

[12] Diabetes Prevention Program Research Group(2002). Reduction in the incidence of type 2 diabetes with lifestyle intervention or metformin. N Engl J Med, , 346, 393-403.

[13] Dragnes, B. T, Larsen, R, Ernstsen, M. H, Mæhre, H, & Elvevoll, E. O. (2009). Impact of processing on the taurine content in processed seafood and their corresponding unprocessed raw materials. Int J Food Sci Nutr, , 60(2), 143-152.

[14] ENSMinisterio de Salud Chile. Encuesta Nacional, htpp:www.minsal.cl/portal/url/page/minsalcl/g_home/home.html, 2009-2010.

[15] FitzGerald RO`Cuinn G, (2006). Enzymatic debittering of food protein hydrolysates. Biotechnol Adv, , 24, 234-237.

[16] Fritsche, K, & Johnston, P. (1988). Rapid autoxidation of fish oil in diets without added antioxidants. J Nutrition, , 118-425.

[17] Fujita, H, & Yoshikawa, M. (1999). LKPNM: a prodrug-type ACE-inhibitory peptide derived from fish protein. Immunopharmacology, 44(1-2): 123-127.

[18] Galardy, R, Podhasky, P, & Olson, K. R. (1984). Angiotensin-converting enzyme activity in tissues of the rainbow trout. J Exp Zool, , 230(1), 155-158.

[19] González-torres, M, Betancourt-rule, M, & Ortiz, R. (2000). Daño oxidativo y antioxidantes. Bioquímica, , 25, 3-9.

[20] Gramza, A, & Korczak, J. (2005). Tea constituents (Camellia sinensis L.) as antioxidants in lipid systems. Trends in Food Science & Technology, , 16, 351-358.

[21] Guadix, A, Guadix, E, Páez-dueñas, M, González-tello, P, & Camacho, F. (2000). Procesos tecnológicos y métodos de control en la hidrólisis de proteínas. Ars Pharmaceutica, , 40, 79-89.

[22] Hoyle, N. T, & Merritt, J. H. (1994). Quality of Fish Protein Hydrolysates from Herring (Clupeaharengus). J Food Sci, , 59, 76-80.

[23] Iglesias de la Cruz CRuiz-Torres P, García del Moral R, Rodríguez-Puyol M, Rodríguez-Puyol D, (2000). Age-related progressive renal fibrosis in rats and its prevention with ACE inhibitors and taurine. Am J Physiol Renal Physiol, 278: FF129., 122.

[24] Iso, H, Date, C, Wakai, K, Fukui, M, & Tamakoshi, A. and the JACC Study Group, (2006). The relationship between green tea intake and type 2 diabetes in Japanese adults. Ann Inter Med, , 144, 554-562.

[25] Kim, S. W, Rogers, Q. R, & Morris, J. G. (1996). Maillard reaction products in purified diets induce taurine depletion in cats which is reversed by antibiotics. J Nutr, , 126(1), 195-201.

[26] Kohama, Y, Kuroda, T, Itoh, S, & Mimura, T. (1996). Tuna muscle peptide, PTHIKWGD, inhibits leukocyte-mediated injury and leukocyte adhesion to cultured endothelial cells. Biol Pharm Bull, , 19(1), 139-41.

[27] Kondo, K, Iwamoto, T, Hooda, K, Kamiyama, M, Hirano, R, Kidou, T, Matsumoto, A, Watanabe, S, & Itakura, H. (2000). Inhibition of low-density lipoprotein oxidation by fish protein and antioxidants. XIIth International Symposium on Atherosclerosis, Abstract W12: 113. June Stockholm, Sweden.(TuP18), 25-29.

[28] Kristinsson, H. G, & Rasco, B. A. (2000). Fish protein hydrolysates: production, biochemical, and functional properties, Crit Rev Food Sci Nutr, , 40, 43-81.

[29] Liaset, B, Julshamn, K, & Espe, M. (2003). Chemical composition and theoretical nutritional evaluation of the produced fractions from enzyme hydrolysis of salmon frames with Protamex. Process Biochemistry, , 38, 1747-1759.

[30] Liceaga-gesualdo, A, & Li-chan, E. (1999). Functional properties of fish protein hydrolysate from herring," J Food Sci, , 64-1000.

[31] Lindström, J, Ilanne-parikka, P, Peltonen, M, Aunola, S, Eriksson, J, & Hemio, K. (2006). Sustained reduction in the incidence of type 2 diabetes by lifestyle intervention: follow-up of the Finnish Diabetes Prevention Study. Lancet, , 368, 1673-1679.

[32] Lindström, J, & Tuomilehto, J. (2003). The Diabetes Risk Score. A practical tool to predict type 2 diabetes risk. Diabetes Care, , 26, 725-731.

[33] Mendis, E, Rajapakse, N, & Kim, S. (2005). Antioxidant properties of a radical-scavenging peptide purified from enzymatically prepared fish skin gelatin hydrolysate. J Agric Food Chem, , 53, 581-587.

[34] Nittynen, L, Nurminen, M. L, Korpela, R, & Vapaatalo, H. (1999). Role of arginine, taurine and homocysteine in cardiovascular diseases. Ann Med, , 31(5), 318-326.

[35] Palic, A, & Lucan, Ž. (1995). Antioxidative Effect of 'Herbalox' on Edible Oils. Lipid/Fett, , 97, 379-381.

[36] Redsalud(2006). www.redsalud.gov.cl/archivos/guiasges/diabetesGES.pdf   http://www.fao.org/docrep/016/i3027e/i3027e03.pdf

[37] Rizzo, M. R, Abbatecola, A. M, Barbieri, M, et al. (2008). Evidence for anti-inflammatory effects of combined administration of vitamin E and C in older persons with impaired fasting glucose: impact on insulin action. J Am Coll Nutr, , 27, 505-11.

[38] Sathivel, S, & Smiley, S. (2005). Functional and nutritional properties of red salmon enzymatic hydrolysates. Journal of Food, , 70, 401-406.

[39] Smith, A, & Munro, N. D. (2009). A holistic approach to examining ancient agriculture. Curr Anthropol, , 50, 925-936.

[40] Valenzuela, A, Sanhueza, J, & Nieto, S. (2003). Natural antioxidants in functional foods: from food safety to health benefits. Grasas y aceites, , 104, 754-760.

[41] Van Dam, R, Willett, W, Manson, J, & Hu, F. (2006). Coffee, caffeine, and risk of type 2 diabetes. Diabetes Care, , 29, 398-403.

[42] Vioque, J, & Millán, F. (2005). Los hidrolizados proteicos en alimentación: Suplementos alimenticios de gran calidad funcional y nutricional. Agro CSIC, , 2-8.

[43] Wanasundara, U, & Shahidi, F. (1998). Antioxidant and pro-oxidant activity of green tea extracts in marine oils. Food Chemistry, , 63, 335-342.

[44] World Health Organization Prevalence of Diabetes(2010). htpp://www.who:int/diabetes/facts/world:figures/en/indexx2.html

[45] Yu, H-H, Liu, X, Xing, R, Liu, S, Guo, Z, Wang, P, Li, C, & Li, P. (2006). In vitro determination of antioxidant activity of proteins from jellyfish. Food Chemistry, , 95, 123-130.

Chapter 5

Pharmacological Treatments for Type 2 Diabetes

Roberto Pontarolo,
Andréia Cristina Conegero Sanches, Astrid Wiens,
Helena Hiemisch Lobo Borba, Luana Lenzi and
Suelem Tavares da Silva Penteado

Additional information is available at the end of the chapter

1. Introduction

Type 2 diabetes mellitus (T2DM) results from relative defects in insulin secretion and action. T2DM may be associated with metabolic syndrome, and it is characterized by insulin resistance, android obesity, dyslipidemia and hypertension. Furthermore, it is responsible for increased morbidity and mortality related to cardiovascular diseases.

In Latin America, diabetes is a major health problem, where the prevalence has reached more than 19 million people [1], many of whom are at the productive age for work. This phenomenon has resulted in an increased burden on social security, thereby fueling the continuation of the vicious cycle of poverty and social exclusion.

In terms of morbidity, diabetes mellitus currently represents one of the major chronic diseases affecting people today, including individuals in countries at all stages of economic and social development. Even developed countries, which, despite scientific advances and easy access to health care, are affected by the increasing prevalence of diabetes. Thus, it is assumed that interventions aimed at preventing this disease, such as physical activity and diet, are underutilized [2].

The relevance of diabetes has increased in recent decades as a result of various factors, such as a high urbanization rate, increased life expectancy, industrialization, hypercaloric diets rich in carbohydrates, displacement of populations to urban areas, changes in lifestyle, physical inactivity and obesity. It is estimated that by 2020, two-thirds of the disease burden will be attributed to chronic, noncommunicable diseases [3]. High-calorie diets and sedentary lifestyles are the major factors contributing to the increased prevalence of obesity, representing additional major risk factors for T2DM [4].

Diabetes is the seventh leading cause of death in the United States. Among adults diagnosed with either type 1 or type 2 diabetes,12 percent take insulin only, 14 percent take both insulin and oral medication, 58 percent take oral medication only, and 16 percent do not take either insulin or oral medication [5].

The treatment of diabetes is aimed predominantly at glycemic control. The treatment objectives are to relieve the symptoms, improve the quality of life, prevent acute and chronic complications, reduce mortality and treat the disease. The basic strategies for treatment and disease control of type 1 and 2 diabetes consist primarily of a specific diet, physical activity and the appropriate use of medication (oral agents and / or insulin). The outcome of the treatment depends on providing diabetic patients with education and ensuring that they adopt specific behavioral measures and practices.

Currently, there is a tendency to use unconventional measures of care for patients with chronic diseases, such as methods involving nonpharmacological treatment [6], emphasizing continued practice and frequent daily exercise and walks. These approaches also emphasize proper nutrition, which is now regarded more as a benefit than as a punishment. The use of medications is indicated for T2DM, together with diet and increased physical activity [7, 8].

Because it is not always possible to establish a full behavioral change in the high-risk population, and even trying to improve the prevention of T2DM can be difficult, a number of drugs have been tested with the intention of preventing this disease. Several drugs have been used, and some of the key studies are summarized here, including drugs such as oral anti-diabetic agents and other oral medications.

In obese patients with T2DM, the priority is weight loss. If glycemic control is not achieved after 4 to 6 weeks, drugs that sensitize the action of insulin (biguanide and thiazolidinedione) may be indicated, either in combination or not with anti-obesity drugs. If satisfactory glycemic control is not achieved, drugs that reduce the intestinal absorption of glucose (acarbose or miglitol) or that enhance insulin secretion (sulfonylurea, repaglinide or netaglinida) may be used.

In type 2 diabetic normal weight or overweight (body mass index <30 kg/m^2) individuals, sulfonylureas, repaglinide or nateglinide can be tried initially. If adequate glycemic control is not achieved after 2 to 4 weeks, biguanide, thiazolidinedione or an inhibitor of intestinal absorption of glucose can be added [7, 8].

Often, the effectiveness of the chosen pharmacological treatment cannot be predicted. Pharmacotherapeutic failure or undesired effects that lead to other health problems, such as adverse reactions and toxicities, may arise. These events are regarded as a negative outcomes associated with the medication use.

In some cases, negative results associated with the use of a medication are inevitable, as in the case of some adverse reactions. However, negative reactions can sometimes be avoided, such as those that result from the inappropriate use of a drug or problems with the monitoring of a drug's effects. The occurrence of these avoidable outcomes could be reduced by adequate follow-up of patients [9].

Non-effective treatment of T2DM leads to a significant increase in the values of glycated hemoglobin, which leads to a decreased quality of life for patients and a significant economic impact [10, 11]. The consequences of diabetes on health systems reflect only a fraction of the damage that is caused to individuals, their families and society.

In recent years, great progress in the treatment of T2DM has been observed. Different classes of drugs are used for this purpose, including analog and human insulin, drugs that act by reducing insulin resistance (biguanides and thiazolidinediones), secretagogues and their analogs (sulfonylureas, metglinides, inhibitors of DPP-4 or GLP-1 agonists) and drugs that reduce the rate of degradation of carbohydrates (alfaglicosidase inhibitors). Some treatments have been used for several decades, such as human insulin, which was first isolated in the 1930s. Other drugs have been developed over the last century, including metformin, which is the most used oral antidiabetic in the U.S. today, and liraglutide, an analog of GLP-1.

The current treatments aim to reduce insulin resistance and maintain adequate glycemic control to prevent or reduce microvascular and macrovascular complications by improving the function of the pancreatic beta cells through interventions involving diet, exercise, oral hypoglycemic agents, anti-hyperglycemic agents and / or anti-obesity drugs. There are currently several types of treatments, which may be used alone or in combination.

Among the class of biguanides, which sensitize the action of insulin, are metformin and phenformin. Metformin is used more frequently than phenformin and has fewer side effects (diarrhea, metallic taste and nausea - which may decrease with continued use). Among the advantages of this class of drugs is its anorectic effect, which aids in weight loss, and the fact that it does not cause hypoglycemia (it does not stimulate insulin secretion).

In the United States and some European countries, other classes of antidiabetic thiazolidine-dione derivatives are available, such as rosiglitazone and pioglitazone, which act by increasing the sensitivity of the liver, muscles and adipocytes to insulin, resulting in a decrease in peripheral resistance. The use of troglitazone, which belongs to this therapeutic class, was suspended due to hepatotoxicity. Rosiglitazone is more potent and has lower liver toxicity and fewer interactions with other drugs because it does not induce metabolism by cytochrome P450 (CYP) 3A4. The side effects include upper respiratory tract infections, headache, elevated transaminases, edema, weight gain and anemia. Pioglitazone is also associated with less liver toxicity and has the same mechanism of action and side effects as rosiglitazone. However, pioglitazone interacts with some medications.

The competitive alpha-glucosidase inhibitors, such as acarbose, miglitol and voglibose, act as antagonists of sucrase and amylase, and they also decrease the intestinal absorption of glucose. The most frequent side effects of alpha-glucosidase inhibitors are bloating, diarrhea, abdominal pain and elevated transaminases, and they are contraindicated in cases of inflammatory bowel disease, pregnancy and lactation, hepatic or renal impairment.

Another class of drugs used to treat T2DM is the class of sulfonylureas, including chlorpropamide (first generation), glibenclamide, gliclazide and glipizide (the second generation) and glimepiride (third generation). These drugs act as insulin secretagogues, and the side effects are hypoglycaemia, hematological (leukopenia, agranulocytosis, thrombocytopenia and hemolytic anemia) and gastrointestinal (nausea, vomiting, more rarely cholestatic jaundice) complications and allergic reactions. They may also cause an increase in weight as a result of binding to the plasma proteins, and their effects can be enhanced by the use of other drugs concomitantly, causing hypoglycemia.

Additional insulin secretagogues include repaglinide, nateglinide and meglitinida. Derivatives of benzoic acid and the amino acid D-phenylalanine increase insulin secretion through an action similar to that of the sulfonylureas. Due to their rapid absorption, this action begins approximately 30 minutes after administration. These drugs do not have interactions with other medications and are not contraindicated during pregnancy, lactation or in the presence of other pathologies.

In many diabetic patients, a hypocaloric diet aimed at weight reduction alone is able to control glucose levels. The anti-obesity effects of catecholaminergic (amfepramone, fenproporex, mazindol), serotonergic (fluoxetine, sertraline) and mixed action catecholaminergic and serotonergic (such as sibutramine) drugs that affect appetite and the induction of satiety may be used. In addition to these, orlistat or tetrahydrolipstatin, which inhibit intestinal lipase and fat absorption, may allow a reduction of the dose of hypoglycemic medications.

The use of insulin in the treatment of T2DM reverses diabetes symptoms and may be used in those with severe hyperglycemia with ketonemia or ketonuria, newly diagnosed patients, or in diabetics who do not respond to treatment with diet, exercise and / or treatments with oral hypoglycemic agents with anti-hyperglycemic or insulin-sensitizing action. Initially, human insulin in association with porcine insulin and regular or single insulin were used. There is a high chance of developing hypoglycemia as a result of the use of interprandial insulin analogous, which have faster action than human insulin. Currently, several types of insulin analogs have been synthesized: lispro, aspart and glargine. These analogs differ in their speed of action and duration of effect due to structural changes in the position of the amino acid chains of insulin. There are multiple options for the rout of administration, and they can be used in combination with oral hypoglycemic agents.

New drugs for the treatment of diabetes are emerging, making multiple therapeutic options possible. Furthermore, the use of insulin by inhalation has been studied to reduce the difficulties associated with subcutaneous administration.

The aim of this chapter was to evaluate all of the available treatments for T2DM, their mechanisms of action and side effects, and also to describe the emerging drugs and trends that are anticipated in the coming years. A better understanding of the mechanisms of action of drugs and the adverse reactions associated with them is important for health professionals and caregivers of patients with T2DM.

2. Treatments

2.1. Biguanides

Metformin and phenformin are oral antidiabetic drugs of the biguanide class. Metformin is the drug of choice for treatment of adults with T2DM due to its low frequency of side effects. It is currently used by nearly one-third of diabetic patients in Italy and is prescribed in the U.S. (> 40 m million prescriptions in 2008). Phenformin is no longer marketed in many countries, although it is still available in Italy [12, 13].

Both metformin and phenformin facilitate weight loss in obese nondiabetic patients without appreciably reducing glucose levels in the blood of such individuals. This weight loss is attributed to the anorectic effect and the slight reduction in the gastrointestinal absorption of carbohydrates [14].

2.1.1. Metformin

Metformin is marketed in tablets of 500 or 850 mg, and the maximum dose is 2.5 g/day, although there are no reports in the literature on the use of metformin at doses up to 3 g when administered after meals to minimize gastrointestinal side effects [15]. It has been reported that this drug increases the number and improves the affinity of insulin receptors in adipocytes and muscle. In the muscle, metformin increases glucose uptake by 15 to 40% and stimulates glycogenolysis. In adipocytes, metformin inhibits lipolysis and the availability of free fatty acids (FFA). Moreover, metformin improves insulin action in the liver, decreasing hepatic production of glucose by 10 to 30% and, at the cellular level, it increases the tyrosine kinase activity of the insulin receptor, stimulating translocation of GLUT4 and the activity of glycogen synthase [16].

The use of metformin also improves the lipid profile, resulting in a decrease in the triglyceride levels by 20 to 25%, a decrease in LDL-cholesterol by as much as 10%, an increase in HDL-cholesterol by 17%, and a decrease in the level of factor plasminogen activator inhibitor (PAI-1) by 20-30 %. Insulin secretion in response to stimuli may remain unchanged or decrease as a result of the anorectic effect, which helps with weight loss. In addition to being associated with weight reduction, its effectiveness in glycemic control is similar to that of sulfonylurea [17]. Another advantage of metformin is that it does not induce hypoglycemia or stimulate insulin secretion [18].

The isolated use of metformin in T2DM lowers blood glucose by approximately 25%, or 60 to 70 mg / dl, and glycosylated hemoglobin is reduced by 1.5 to 2% [16]. The intensive glucose control resulting from the use of metformin significantly decreases the risk of cardiovascular disease and mortality related to diabetes and patients presented less weight gain compared to other medications including insulin. Metformin also avoids the inconvenience of hypoglycemia induced by treatment with insulin or sulfonylureas [19].

Metformin is absorbed in the intestine and excreted by the kidneys. It is minimally metabolized by the liver, has a low affinity for mitochondrial membranes, and it does not interfere with oxidative phosphorylation. Metformin is indicated as a monotherapy in obese diabetic or glucose intolerant patients. Approximately 5 to 10% of patients each year will not have an appropriate response to the drug. In these cases, to achieve satisfactory control, metformin can be used in combination with sulfonylureas, acarbose, thiazolidinedione, repaglinide and / or insulin [7, 20-24].

The most frequent side effects are diarrhea (15%), a metallic taste and nausea, and these often decrease with continued use of the medication. The occurrence of lactic acidosis is rare (0.03 to 0.4 / 1000/year), occurring most often in people who have a contraindication to metformin, such as chronic liver disease (elevated transaminase 2 to 3 times normal values), heart failure, respiratory or renal failure (creatinine clearance <70 ml / min or serum creatinine ≥ 1.5 mg / dl). Metformin is not advisable for use in people over age 80, pregnant women, infants or alcoholics. In patients with proteinuria or those who are subjected to radiological examination containing iodine, it is prudent to provide adequate hydration and discontinue the medication a few days before [18]. Metformin shows synergistic effects with cimetidine and may decrease the absorption of vitamin B12 [15].

2.1.2. Phenformin

Phenformin presents a hypoglycemic action based on its insulin-sensitizing properties, similar to metformin. Approximately 30% of phenformin has hepatic metabolism and shows a high affinity for mitochondrial membranes, and it may also interfere with oxidative phosphorylation [18].

Due to its greater propensity to cause serious and fatal adverse events such as lactic acidosis, this drug was withdrawn from clinical practice in the 1970s. These effects are attributed to inhibition of Complex I of the mitochondrial respiratory chain. However, though no longer in clinical use, phenformin remains a widely used research tool to help delineate the cellular and molecular mechanisms that underlie the action of biguanides [25].

2.2. Thiazolidinediones

The thiazolidinediones (TZD) are popularly known as glitazones. Among the representatives of TZD are troglitazone (withdrawn from the market due to liver toxicity), rosiglitazone and pioglitazone (second generation thiazolidinediones).

Widely used in the treatment of T2DM, these drugs exert their effect by increasing and sensitizing insulin action in the liver, muscle and fat cells, decreasing peripheral resistance. They activate the intracellular nuclear receptors (PPAR-gamma, peroxisome proliferator activated receptor), which regulate the expression of genes involved in the metabolism of glucose and lipids, genes that are responsible for glucose uptake mediated by insulin in the peripheral tissues and genes that participated in the differentiation of preadipocytes into adipocytes. Moreover, these drugs inhibit peripheral lipolysis in adipocytes and assist in reducing the levels of free fatty acids and visceral adiposity, resulting in improvement of glycemic and metabolic parameters in these patients. They show good results in maintaining long-term glycemic control compared with other therapeutic options such as sulfonylureas and metformin [26-28].

Thiazolidinediones decrease glucose levels by approximately 20%, but no increase insulin secretion is observed. These drugs inhibit oxidation of long chain fatty acids in the liver, and they decrease gluconeogenesis and the availability of free fatty acids. Although they induce a decrease of triglycerides by 15 to 20% and an increase of HDL-cholesterol of 5 to 10%, the total cholesterol and LDL-cholesterol levels may not change or they may increase by 10 to 15% [18]. When compared to metformin, it has been observed that troglitazone has a greater potentiating effect for peripheral insulin action and less of an effect for reducing the hepatic glucose output. The association of thiazolidinedione with metformin is interesting because these drugs have additive effects [22].

Thiazolidinediones also increase the expression of the glucose transporter (GLUT4) and lipoprotein lipase, and they reduce the expression of leptin and tumor necrosis factor (TNF-alpha). These results make this drug class the most widely prescribed for the treatment of T2DM [18, 29].

Side effects occur in less than 5% of patients, consisting of upper respiratory tract infections, headache, elevated transaminases, edema, weight gain and anemia. Hypoglycemia can occur when the use of thiazolidinediones is concomitant with secretagogues or insulin. Their use is contraindicated in children, pregnant women, or in individuals with elevated transaminase levels that are 2-3 times the values of reference [18].

2.2.1. Troglitazone

In mice subjected to arterial injury, troglitazone inhibited the growth of vascular smooth muscle cells and intimal hyperplasia, suggesting that thiazolidinediones decrease the progression of atherosclerosis. In diabetic patients treated with troglitazone, decreases were observed in platelet aggregation, factor plasminogen activator inhibitor (PAI-1) and blood pressure levels. These multiple effects strengthen its indication for the treatment of metabolic syndrome. However, caution is recommended with the indication because of the possibility of hepatic complications, including reports of fatalities associated with the use of troglitazone. Additionally, this drug should be administered with caution in cardiac patients due to the possibility of edema [18, 30, 31].

2.2.2. Pioglitazone

Pioglitazone can be used as monotherapy or in combination with metformin, which has anti-hyperglycemic effects, or with sulfonylurea, meglitinida, or even insulin, especially in diabetic patients with metabolic syndrome. The dose varies from 15 to 45 mg, and it may be administered once a day. This drug displays mechanism of action and similar side effects to rosiglitazone, and it causes less liver toxicity than troglitazone. However, pioglitazone may interact with other drugs metabolized by P450 enzymes through changing their serum levels. An example is a decrease by approximately 30% of the contraceptive effect of ethinyl estradiol and norethindrone. Accordingly, the dose of the contraceptive must be increased in diabetic women who do not wish to become pregnant. The pharmacokinetics of pioglitazone are not altered by mild to moderate renal insufficiency [32].

2.2.3. Rosiglitazone

Rosiglitazone is more potent and has lower hepatotoxicity than troglitazone. Furthermore, it stimulates metabolism by cytochrome P450 (CYP) 3A4 without interacting with oral contraceptives, digoxin, ranitidine or nifedipine. Rosiglitazone dosage varies from 4 to 8 mg, and it may be given once a day. Similar to pioglitazone, rosiglitazone's pharmacokinetics are not altered by mild to moderate renal insufficiency, and dose modification is not required [33].

Recently published safety data prompted concerns about a possible association between the chronic use of rosiglitazone and an increased risk of cardiovascular events, leading to some parsimony in the use of TZDs in clinical practice. Furthermore, studies have recently shown bone loss and increased fracture among users of these medications in [27, 29, 34].

2.3. Alpha-glucosidase inhibitors

The competitive inhibitors of alpha-glucosidase, such as acarbose, miglitol and voglibose, act as enzymatic antagonists of oligosaccharide (e.g. amylase, maltase and sucrase) and decrease the intestinal absorption of glucose, particularly postprandial absorption, thereby modulating the insulin secretion [35]. These inhibitors present the advantage of lowering the incidence of cardiovascular events, and they have no systemic absorption [36].

More specifically, alpha-glucosidase is inhibited competitively, and its availability for oligosaccharides derived from the diet is reduced. Thus, the formation of monosaccharide decreases, and less insulin is required for metabolism, which leads to a reduction of glucose (because it is not absorbed) as well as postprandial insulin-induced increases [37]. These effects reflect a significant decrease in glycated hemoglobin [38, 39], which is more evident in highly hyperglycemic patients. Hyperglycemia in patients with mild or moderate glycemic control is less common than in those using other oral antidiabetic agents. In such cases, competitive inhibitors of alpha-glucosidase can be used in combination with insulin or any other oral hypoglycemic agents.

2.3.1. Acarbose

Acarbose has microbial origin and is structurally similar to natural oligosaccharides, having an affinity 104-105 times higher than drugs of the same class of alpha-glucosidases. With regard to the pharmacokinetic aspects, acarbose is poorly absorbed in the intestine (less than 2%). The products produced by bacterial enzymes cleave acarbose, yielding intermediate 4-metipiro-galol, which is conjugated and excreted as sulfates or glucuronidate [39].

In a prospective, randomized, double-blind, placebo-controlled trial [40], there was a satisfactory control of fasting and postprandial glucose with acarbose in T2DM. In a multicenter, randomized, double-blind, placebo-controlled clinical trial [41] conducted in patients with T2DM who were subjected to a specific diet and use of insulin, the patients showed decreased levels of blood glucose and glycated hemoglobin as well as a reduced daily requirement for insulin.

In a systematic review [42], it was concluded that acarbose inhibits postprandial hyperglycemia by lowering insulin levels after a glucose overload. However, it presents no advantages with respect to corporal weight or lipid metabolism, and there are no statistically significant effects on mortality, morbidity and quality of life in patients with T2DM. Compared with placebo, acarbose reduces HbA1c and fasting plasma glucose and postprandial glucose. Compared with sulfonylureas, it reduces glycemic control and has major adverse effects, particularly gastrointestinal.

2.3.2. Voglibose

Voglibose also has a microbial origin, and only 3-5% of the drug is absorbed at the intestinal level. It is a potent inhibitor of alpha-glucosidase, but it is weaker than acarbose in the inhibition of sucrase and has little effect on pancreatic alpha-amylase [39].

2.3.3. Miglitol

Miglitol has a synthetic origin. It is absorbed rapidly through a transport mechanism in the jejunum that is partly identical to glucose, and it is quantitatively excreted unchanged by the kidney. Miglitol differs from acarbose, as it does not inhibit alpha-amylase, but rather it inhibits intestinal isomaltase [39].

The most frequent side effects of alpha-glucosidase inhibitors are seen at the intestinal level: flatulence, diarrhea, abdominal pain and elevated transaminases. The occurrence of hypoglycemia and an increase in body weight are rare because the agent does not stimulate insulin release or hypersecretion. These effects are only observed when miglitol is combined with other therapies. Its use is contraindicated in cases of inflammatory bowel disease, pregnancy and lactation, and hepatic or renal impairment.

2.4. Sulfonylureas

Another class of drugs used in the treatment of T2DM is the class of sulfonylureas, chlorpropamide and tolbultamide (first generation), glibenclamide, glipizide and gliclazide (second generation) and glimepiride (third generation). This class was introduced commercially in the 1950s and has since been recognized as first-line therapy and as a monotherapy or in combination [43]. The sulfonylureas are the drugs of choice for type 2 diabetics who do not benefit exclusively from diet and exercise [44].

These drugs act as insulin secretagogues and exert their main action on islet B cells, stimulating insulin secretion and thereby reducing the plasma glucose concentration [45]. The mechanism of action involves binding of the drug to a subunit of the ATP-sensitive potassium channels in the plasma membranes of B cells. The channels are closed, leading to a change in the membrane voltage, calcium influx and exocytosis of insulin granules [46, 47].

The basal secretion and insulin secretory response to various stimuli are intensified in the early days of treatment with sulfonylureas. With longer-term treatment, insulin secretion continues to increase, and tissue sensitivity to insulin also improves by an unknown mechanism [45].

The sulphonylureas are well absorbed after oral administration, and most reach peak plasma concentrations in 2-4 hours. The duration of the effect varies. All of these drugs bind tightly to plasma albumin and are involved in interactions with other drugs (e.g., salicylates and sulfonamides) such that there is competition for binding sites. The sulfonylureas (or their active metabolites) are mostly excreted in the urine; thus, their action is increased in elderly patients or those with renal disease [45].

2.4.1. First-generation sulfonylureas

The action of chlorpropamide and tolbutamide is long lasting, with substantial excretion in urine. Therefore, these drugs can cause severe hypoglycemia in elderly patients where there is a progressive decline in glomerular filtration. They cause flushing after alcohol consumption and exert similar effects to the diuretic hormone on the distal nephron, producing hyponatremia and water intoxication [45].

2.4.2. Second-generation sulfonylureas

The second-generation sulfonylureas (glibenclamide, glipizide and gliclazide) are more potent, but their hypoglycemic effects are not much greater, and failure to control blood glucose is as commonly observed as that with tolbutamide. All of these drugs contain the sulfonylurea molecule, but different substitutions result in pharmacokinetic differences, and thus differences in the duration of action. Glibenclamide should be avoided in the elderly and in patients with mild renal impairment because of the risk of hypoglycemia, as several of its metabolites are excreted in the urine and are moderately active [45].

The sulfonylureas cross the placenta and stimulate insulin release by fetal B cells, causing severe hypoglycemia at birth. Consequently, their use is contraindicated during pregnancy, and gestational diabetes is treated by diet supplemented where necessary with insulin [45].

In general, sulfonylureas are well tolerated. The observed side effects are hypoglycemia, hematological (leukopenia, agranulocytosis, thrombocytopenia, and hemolytic anemia) and gastrointestinal (nausea, vomiting, more rarely cholestatic jaundice) problems and allergic reactions. Sulfonylureas may also cause weight gain, and binding to plasma proteins can be potentiated by other drugs used concomitantly, causing hypoglycemia. This condition is the most worrisome adverse event observed and may be prolonged, which can have severe consequences in elderly patients, patients treated with multiple drugs and those with impaired renal function. Moreover, sulfonylureas stimulate appetite and can occasionally cause allergic rashes and bone marrow injury [45].

2.4.3. Glimepiride

The United States Food and Drug Administration (FDA) approved glimepiride in 1995 for the treatment of T2DM alone and in combination with metformin or insulin. It has prolonged action, lasting over 24 hours. Glimepiride has advantages with respect to its clinical and pharmacological profile, and it has also been shown to cause a lower incidence of severe hypoglycemia compared to other representatives of their class [48, 49].

Regarding hypoglycemia, the findings observed in some studies differ. In a systematic review and meta-analysis [50], we concluded that glimepiride caused more hypoglycemia compared to other sulfonylureas, and even more than other secretagogues. In other studies, the long-acting sulfonylureas, such as chlorpropamide and glibenclamide, have been shown to be more likely to cause hypoglycemia [51-53]. In a UK survey, the rate of diagnosis of hypoglycemia was higher for glibenclamide compared to other representatives of the same class [51].

With regard to weight gain, in the United Kingdom Prospective Diabetes Study (UKPDS), the mean weight change after 10 years of follow up ranged from a minimum of 1.7 kg as a result of glibenclamide use to a maximum 2.6 kg with chlorpropamide use [19]. Glimepiride was claimed to be at least neutral with respect to body weight, and weight reduction has been observed by some authors [54, 55].

Sulfonylureas have different cross reactivities with cardiovascular ATP-dependent potassium channels. The closing of these channels by ischemic preconditioning can lead to cardiovascular mortality [56].

Several compounds increase the hypoglycemic effect of sulfonylureas, and several of these interactions are potentially important from a clinical standpoint. The non-steroidal anti-inflammatory agents (including azapropazone, phenylbutazone and salicylates), coumarin, some uricosuric agents (e.g., sulfinpyrazone), alcohol, monoamine oxidase inhibitors, some antibacterials (including sulfonamides, and chloramphenicol trimethropim) and some antifungal agents (including miconazole and possibelmente, fluconazole) produce severe hypoglycemia when administered with sulfonylureas. The probable basis for these interactions is the competition for metabolizing enzymes, but interference in the plasma protein binding or excretion may also exert some effect. The agents that reduce the action of sulfonylureas include diuretics (thiazides and loop diuretics) and corticosteroids [45].

2.5. Glinides

Other insulin secretagogues drugs include repaglinide, nateglinide and mitiglinide. Derivatives of benzoic acid and the amino acid D-phenylalanine increase insulin secretion through an action similar to the sulfonylureas. Due to their rapid absorption, the action begins approximately 30 minutes after administration. These drugs have no interactions with other medication and are not contraindicated in pregnancy, lactation or in the presence of other pathologies

Repaglinide and nateglinide are insulin secretagogues with short action, with a half-life equivalent to 1 hour for the repaglinide and 1.5 h for nateglinide. Both of these secretagogues act by triggering an insulin peak during the postprandial period when administered before meals [57].

2.5.1. Repaglinide

Repaglinide ((S) - (+)-2-ethoxy-4-[2 - (3-methyl-1-[2 - (piperidin-1-yl) phenyl] Butylamino)-2-oxoethyl] benzoic acid) was the first representative of the class of glinides, which differs from other classes of anti-hyperglycemic drugs due to its distinct molecular structure, mechanism of action and mechanism excretion [58].

This drug acts as a short-acting insulin secretagogue that targets the postprandial-released glucose. It significantly reduces the levels of plasma glucose in individuals with T2DM [59].

The mechanism of action of repaglinide involves blocking potassium efflux from pancreatic β cells. This action depolarizes the cells by opening voltage-gated calcium channels. This process results in increased calcium influx into the B cells, which stimulates the exocytosis of insulin-containing secretory granules [60, 61]. Regarding the pharmacokinetics, this drug has rapid absorption and rapid elimination, with a plasma half-life of up to 1 hour [61]. Repaglinide is primarily metabolized in the liver, and 90% of the drug is excreted through the gut and 8% through the urine [62]. Because the action of this drug is rapid and the time of effect is relatively short, it carries a low risk of hypoglycemia [63]. Repaglinide may be used as a monotherapy or in combination with other antidiabetic agents, such as metformin and glitazone [62].

2.5.2. Nateglinide

Nateglinide (3-phenyl-2-[(4-propan-2-ylcyclohexanecarbonyl) amino] propanoic acid) as well as repaglinide acts by inhibiting potassium channels that are sensitive to ATP, causing depolarization of the plasma membrane of the β cell. This processes culminates in the influx of calcium ions into the cell and subsequent insulin secretion [64]. Nateglinide is thus an insulinotropic agent that is capable of restoring the physiological pattern of insulin secretion, which is not regulated in diabetic patients [65].

Potassium channels are known to be ATP-dependent in cardiac cells as well as in pancreatic β cells. Thus, a reasonable degree of concern exists regarding the influence of therapeutic agents that act on these channels on heart function. Nateglinide has a high selectivity for pancreatic potassium channels and is more reliable in relation to repaglinide and glibenclamide with regard to the possible onset of cardiovascular events [65].

Nateglinide induces rapid and transient insulin secretion in a glucose-dependent manner. The response of potassium channels to nateglinide is remarkably lower during periods of euglycemia compared to periods when the glucose levels are high. Thus, the minimum total insulin exposure generated by this drug protects against hypoglycemia attacks, allowing the patient some flexibility regarding the intervals between meals [62].

The effects of nateglinide are specific to prandial insulin release, allowing for the observed reduction in glycated hemoglobin (HbA1c) without the risk of hypoglycemia between meals [65].

With regard to the pharmacokinetic properties, nateglinide is rapidly absorbed, and the peak plasma concentration is reached in 1 hour. The drug metabolism occurs in the liver, and approximately 10% is excreted unchanged via the kidneys [62].

As with repaglinide, nateglinide can be used as a monotherapy or in combination with other agents, such as metformin or glitazone. Both repaglinide and nateglinide have similar efficacy for reducing the fasting blood glucose levels and postprandial plasma glucose, and during early insulin secretion, they contribute to an improvement of insulin sensitivity and pancreatic β cell function. However, repaglinide was shown to be more effective with regard to reducing HbA1c [65].

2.5.3. Mitiglinide

Mitiglinide is also an analogue of the meglitinides, and it has a mechanism of action that has been previously elucidated for other substances [60]. However, mitiglinide is not yet approved by the FDA for the treatment of T2DM.

2.6. Treatment based on the effects of incretin hormones

The use of incretin hormones in the treatment of type 2 diabetes is the subject of extensive investigations that have culminated in the development of new classes of drugs that have been recently approved for the treatment of the disease. The intensification of the action of incretin, especially GLP-1, is the basis of numerous new options for the metabolic control of T2DM.

Incretin mimetics, such as exenatide, as well as inhibitors of the enzyme DPP-4, such as sitagliptin and vildagliptin, have been developed. In general, these agents reduce the blood glucose levels to a level similar to that induced by other oral hypoglycemic agents with minimal risk of hypoglycemia. Furthermore, they have potential preventive effects and may promote disease regression. They may also have possible protective effects and promote growth in pancreatic β cells.

2.7. Antagonists of GLP-1R

2.7.1. Exenatide

Exenatide is an exendin-4 GLP-1 mimetic with ~53% homology to endogenous GLP-1. It is currently approved for use as a monotherapy or in combination with metformin and/or sulphonylureas [66]. Exenatide is administered subcutaneously at a dose of 5 or 10 mg, twice a day. It binds to the GLP-1 receptor and has a longer lasting action because it presents greater resistance to the action of DPP-4 [67, 68].

In phase III studies, exenatide improved glycemic control in patients with type 2 diabetes for whom glycemic control was not achieved with metformin and / or sulfonylurea. These studies were double-blind, placebo-controlled, 30-week trials. The initial HA1c ranged from 8.2% to 8.7% and was reduced by approximately 1% when exenatide was compared with placebo. There was a mean weight loss of approximately 2 Kg. In the clinical trials that have been performed to date, the drop-out rate due to side effects of exenatide was less than 5% [69, 70]

The main adverse effects of exenatide are nausea, vomiting and diarrhea. Most episodes of nausea are mild to moderate and dose dependent, and they decrease in frequency with continued treatment [71].

2.8. GLP-1 analogs

2.8.1. Liraglutide

Liraglutide is a long-acting human GLP-1 analogue that shares 97% amino acid sequence identity with human GLP-1 and is resistant to dipeptidyl peptidase-IV. Native GLP-1 has a short elimination half-life of 1-2 min, whereas liraglutide has a long half-life of approximately 13 hours and can be administered once a day [67, 72]. When administered once daily, liraglutide enables significantly superior glycemic control compared to that obtained with the administration of exenatide 2 times per day and is generally well tolerated [69].

Other GLP-1 analogs, taspoglutide and albiglutide are currently in phase III clinical trials. Albiglutide has a long half-life, allowing administration once per week.

2.9. DPP-4 inhibitors

2.9.1. Vildagliptin

Vildagliptin is a DPP-4 inhibitor that prolongs the activity of endogenous GLP-1. A study that compared vildagliptin with metformin showed a smaller decrease in HA1c after one year with vildagliptin, but fewer gastrointestinal side effects. Comparison of vildagliptin and pioglitazone showed similar reductions in HA1c [73].

Vildagliptin is used in several countries, but it has not been approved by the FDA because of the occurrence of elevated enzyme levels in patients taking higher doses of vildagliptin.

2.9.2. Sitagliptin

Sitagliptin is a DPP-4 inhibitor that was approved by the FDA in October 2006 to improve glycemic control in patients with type 2 diabetes. It is approved for use as a monotherapy or in combination with other oral hypoglycemic agents. It is administered at a dose of 100 mg per day [74]. Treatment with this DPP-4 inhibitor is generally well tolerated. Sitagliptin monotherapy or in combination was shown to have a neutral effect on body weight. The incidence of hypoglycemia and gastrointestinal effects, such as abdominal pain, diarrhea, nausea and vomiting, was not significantly different between the groups treated with sitagliptin and placebo [75].

Sitagliptin displays a relatively low effectiveness in reducing HA1c and plasma glucose compared to other antidiabetic agents that have been utilized clinically for many years. Additionally, sitagliptin does not have beneficial effects beyond its effects on glycemic control, such as reduction in body weight [76].

Alogliptina and saxagliptin are still under investigation, and they have not been approved for use by the FDA.

2.10. Anti-obesity drugs

Many clinical studies have reported the significant influence of excess body fat on metabolic disorders, such as T2DM. Notably, patients with T2DM who are significantly overweight (20% to 40%) have a higher mortality rate compared with patients with the same disease but who are within the proper range of weight. In many diabetic patients, a reduced calorie diet aimed at weight reduction alone is able to control blood glucose levels. However, for these individuals, body weight control is more complicated, both due to a mechanism of disease and for the treatment of disease. Thus, many doctors resort to drugs that are capable of inducing weight loss in patients with metabolic disorders [77].

In patients whose body mass index (BMI) is above 30 kg/m2 or those with morbid conditions associated with overweight for whom non-pharmacological weight loss methods (diet, exercise) have failed, the use of antiobesity drugs is recommended [78]. These drugs may include medications with catecholaminergic action (amfepramone, femproporex, mazindol), serotonergic action (fluoxetine, sertraline) and mixed catecholaminergic and serotonergic action (such as sibutramine), which promote appetite control and induction of satiety. In addition to these drugs, tetrahydrolipstatin or orlistat may be used to inhibit lipase reducing intestinal fat absorption, allowing for a reduction of the dose of the hypoglycemic drug.

Amfepramone (diethylpropion), femproporex and mazindol are amphetamine derivatives. They work by stimulating the central nervous system, prompting the release of noradrenaline in the central and peripheral synapses. Through this mechanism, these drugs cause appetite suppression [79]. Amfepramone has been available in the market for weight loss since the 1960s [80]. It has been demonstrated in clinical trials with animals that mazindol stimulates the consumption of oxygen by increasing the stimulation of noradrenaline in the brown adipose tissue. Through this thermogenic effect, mazindol is capable of inducing weight loss [78].

The anorectic catecholaminergic drugs usually have good gastrointestinal absorption and are able to reach peak plasma levels within 2 hours of administration, and their metabolism is mainly hepatic. The catecholaminergic drugs have serious side effects, such as increased heart rate and blood pressure [78]. Generally, the use of amphetamine derivatives is accompanied by a remarkable pharmacodynamic tolerance, and their anorectic actions over the long term are not known [79].

Catecholaminergic and serotonergic medications have different effects on food intake. The former delay the start of ingestion, and the latter anticipate the completion of food intake [78].

Sibutramine acts by inhibition of noradrenaline and serotonin receptors, elevating the levels of these neurotransmitters in the hypothalamus and brainstem regions associated with energy homeostasis. This mechanism induces satiety and therefore the reduction of food intake. In addition to generating weight loss, sibutramine significantly reduces triglyceride and HDL-cholesterol levels, its therapeutic action may be accompanied by some adverse effects, such as constipation, headache, and insomnia, which are usually mild [81]. However, cardiovascular events associated with the use of this substance, such as an increased heart rate and elevated blood pressure, are of concern [82, 83].

Orlistat is a reversible inhibitor of pancreatic and gastric lipase that induces weight loss by preventing the absorption of a significant amount of fat digested in the intestine [82]. It inactivates fat hydrolyzing, thereby reducing the absorption of calories by the patient [84]. The effect of orlistat on body weight reduction corresponds to benefits for other cardiometabolic parameters, such as blood pressure, waist circumference, and blood glucose. Among the most common adverse side effects of orlistat are diarrhea, flatulence, bloating and dyspepsia [81].

Although the weight loss caused by these drugs is generally not very significant, there is an improvement in insulin sensitivity and glycemic control in overweight patients who use these substances [84]. This effect emphasizes the importance of aid in the pharmacological management of obesity in patients with T2DM and other metabolic disorders; it is insufficient to only change the patient's lifestyle.

2.11. Insulin

The classification of insulin is based on the preparation. Namely, the duration of its action as short-acting, intermediate or basal insulin determines the classification. The latter two are the result of changes in crystalline insulin (short-acting). The addition of protamine and zinc result in Neutral Protamine Hagedorn (NPH) with intermediate and basal action, respectively.

The change in amino acid sequence allowed for the development of insulin analogues. The fast-acting insulin analogues lispro and aspart are available for clinical use and show similar pharmacokinetic and pharmacodynamic properties. The formulations glargine and detemir represent similar groups that may have either basal or long-term action (24 hours) [85].

2.11.1. Short or ultra-rapid-acting insulin

This group includes regular insulin and the analogues lispro, aspart and glulisine.

Regular insulin is usually administered by the subcutaneous route, often in combination with an intermediate-acting or long-duration insulin. Specific buffers are used to prevent crystallization due to its slow infusion. With this type of insulin, the monomers are presented in an associated hexamer form, which reduces the rate of absorption. Generally, regular insulin is indicated for the treatment of diabetic ketoacidosis, and it is also associated with human insulin intermediate-acting or basal analogs before meals [86]. This insulin must be given 30-45 minutes before meals to reduce the postprandial glycemia peak, and the activity lasts between 2 and 4 hours. However, patients tend to apply it at mealtime, which contributes to postprandial hyperglycemia and hypoglycemia in the period between meals because the regular insulin will peak at the time that the food has been metabolized. The first rapid-acting insulin analogue became available in 1996, and other rapid-acting analogs have been developed since. These analogues were produced by different modifications of the chemical structure of the human insulin protein, substituting various amino acids at different positions to shorten the onset and duration of action when compared to regular/ soluble insulin.

Insulin lispro is an analogue of human insulin developed using genetic engineering to reverse the amino acids proline and lysine in positions 28 and 29 of the beta chain, resulting in a sequence of Lys (B28) Pro (B29). This insulin in pharmaceutical preparations with phenol and zinc forms stable hexamers [86]. It has a lower tendency to self-aggregate at the site of subcutaneous injection, it is absorbed faster than regular human insulin, and it mimics the physiological insulin profile in response to a meal. Lispro begins to take effect within 5 - 15 minutes, and the duration of action is 1-2 hours [87]. During the use of these analogs, an additional dose is required in the afternoon to compensate for hyperglycemia that may result from an afternoon snack. There is evidence that compared with regular insulin, lispro insulin reduces the postprandial hyperglycemic peaks as well as the risk of hypoglycemia, especially at night [86].

In insulin aspart, a proline residue is replaced with a negatively charged aspartic acid at position 28 of the beta chain, producing electrical repulsion among the insulin molecules, which reduces their tendency for self-association. In vials or cartridges, the drug is present in the form of hexamers that rapidly dissociate into monomers and dimers in the subcutaneous tissue, ensuring rapid absorption. The pharmacokinetic profile includes the onset of action within 5 - 15 minutes and a duration of action of 1-2 hours [86].

The insulin glulisine is another insulin analogue with ultra-rapid action that is obtained by the exchange of asparagine for lysine at position 3 of the beta chain and lysine for glutamic acid at position 29 of the same chain. To date, there are few studies with glulisine, which seems to be similar to lispro and aspart with regard to its efficacy and the occurrence of hypoglycemic events. Due to its faster absorption, glulisine should be administered 5-10 minutes before a meal, ensuring greater flexibility for the patient and thus improving his/her quality of life. The short half-life reduces the need to eat food 2-3 hours after its administration, which is necessary with regular insulin, for which the greater half-life causes postprandial hypoglycemia. Although chemical structures of glulisine and insulin are different, no significant difference in time or duration of action was reported between them.

2.11.2. Intermediate-acting insulin

NPH insulin was introduced in 1946. It is a suspension of insulin in a complex with zinc and protamine in a phosphate buffer. Generally, a dose is given once a day before breakfast or twice daily. NPH has an absorption peak at approximately 4.6 hours after subcutaneous administration, followed by a steady decline in the level of plasma insulin [88]. This insulin can be mixed with regular insulin in the same syringe to increase patient compliance, especially in the case of children. However, the zinc present in the slow-acting insulin can prolong the effect of regular insulin [86].

The profiles of action of intermediate-acting insulin make them suitable for systems in which basal insulin is given one to three times daily. A rigid daily feeding programming is required, including a relatively fixed schedule for meals and snacks with consistent indices of carbohydrate meals / snacks. The major disadvantages of NPH are the wide variations in the daily timing and duration of the peaks within and between individuals, which, when compared to long-acting analogs, may result in non-optimal metabolic control and an increased risk for nocturnal hypoglycemia. The slow-acting insulin was used for many years as an intermediate-acting insulin with a profile of action similar to that of NPH.

2.11.3. Basal insulin analogs (long-action insulin analogs)

The insulins glargine and detemir belong to a group referred to as long-acting or basal insulin analogs [86].

Insulin detemir is produced by recombinant DNA technology, with expression in *Saccharomyces cerevisiae* followed by chemical modification [89]. A fatty acid (myristic acid) is attached to the lysine at position 29, which binds to circulating albumin, forming a complex that dissociates slowly, thus prolonging the duration of its action [79]. The insulin detemir is soluble at neutral pH; however, it can be mixed with rapid analogs. Insulin detemir has shown potential benefits for body weight, with weight loss or decreased weight gain in adults, in children and in adolescents [90].

Insulin glargine is synthesized by introducing changes into the amino acid chain of human insulin, including a substitution of asparagine with glycine at position A21 and the addition of two arginines at position B30. These changes result in a standard single release from the injection site. That is, this analog precipitates in the subcutaneous tissue, allowing a gradual absorption into the bloodstream [91].

Basal insulin was developed to promote basal levels within 24 hours, and it may be administered once a day or at bedtime. When comparing conventional long-acting insulin with insulin glargine, it can be observed that insulin has a similar profile at a constant concentration without prominent peaks [92]. It has an onset of action between 1 and 2 hours, reaching the plateau of biological action between 4 and 6 hours with termination of the effect between 20 and 24 hours. Due to a slightly acidic pH, glargine cannot be mixed with any other insulin in the same syringe; accordingly, some children complain of a burning sensation at the application site [86]. The timing of administration of glargine seems to have no impact on its efficacy for glycemic control, but the dose should be given at approximately the same time each day to maintain its efficacy as a free insulin peak action. If a dose is omitted, 50% of the daily insulin will be missed on that day.

2.11.4. Inhalable insulin

The benefits of injectable insulin are often limited, considering the difficulty of persuading patients to comply with the requirements for adequate treatment due to the need for multiple injections [93].

Aiming to alleviate this discomfort, the first US-approved inhaled insulin (Exubera ®) Pfizer / Nektar became available in January 2006. This product consisted of a dry powder formulation containing 1-3 g of human insulin administered via a single inhaler dose [94]. A polyethylene glycol inhalable dry powder that releases the equivalent of 3 to 8 UI of short-acting insulin subcutaneously [95] was developed for this product. Although Exubera has demonstrated efficacy and a low risk of hypoglycemia, there was a poor acceptance by the prescriber and the patient, and in April 2008, the first clinical evidence that it may cause cancer emerged, with 6 cases diagnosed with lung cancer. There were also cases of primary lung malignancy in patients who had a history of smoking. Other important aspects include coughing, pulmonary function deterioration and an increase of anti-insulin antibodies [96].

AERx insulin was developed by Aradigm Corporation and Novo Nordisk. This system generates aerosol droplets from liquid insulin. The device guides the user to inhale reproducibly. It also offers the ability to download data related to the patient's insulin use, such as the frequency of inhalation, allowing for the monitoring of the treatment. Because of the experiences reported in the Exubera studies, their studies have been discontinued [97].

Technosphere Insulin (TI) is another system involving inhaled dry powder blends of recombinant human insulin (MannKind Corp.) using a MedTone ® (Pharmaceutical Discovery Corp.) inhaler. This system is currently in phase II clinical research, and the partners have developed a placebo for inhalation, allowing for controlled and double-blind studies in patients with diabetes mellitus [95, 97].

2.11.5. Insulin and cancer risk

Studies report that chronic hyperinsulinemia is associated with the pathogenesis of colon cancer and also with breast, pancreas and endometrium cancer [98]. One possible mechanism that explains this relationship is that insulin resistance and hyperinsulinemia, which are characteristic of diabetic patients, or even increased levels of therapies based on endogenous insulin secretagogues or insulin, may increase the level of growth factor 1 of insulin, which plays an essential role in carcinogenesis [99]. Insulin receptors are present in (pre)-neoplastic cells, and insulin can stimulate growth. Furthermore, these cells may be susceptible to mechanisms that cause insulin resistance, such as subclinical chronic inflammation with increased TNF-alpha, which act as promoters of tumor growth. Obesity is associated with an increased risk of developing cancer due to factors such as the endocrine and metabolic effects and the consequent changes that they induce in the production of peptide and steroid hormones [98]. The results of a meta-analysis published in 2012 reported an increase of 28% in the risk of developing cancer in patients using insulin compared to non-users. Thus, there is growing that we are experiencing a worldwide epidemic of diabetes mellitus due to a large aging population and the increasing number of obese people who develop insulin resistance and hyperinsulinemia, which may further contribute to the number of patients with cancer [99].

The results of recently published meta-analyses indicate that some cancers develop most frequently in patients with diabetes, especially type 2 diabetes, although prostate cancer was shown to be less frequent in men with diabetes. Thus, preventive measures should be encouraged among the population to prevent these diseases [99].

3. Conclusion

Despite the clear benefits of achieving and maintaining glycemic goals and the availability of newer and potentially more effective drugs for the management of T2DM, the number of patients with poor glycemic control has not substantially decreased over the past 10 years.

The progressive nature of T2DM has been a significant challenge for achieving adequate glycemic control. The inability of classical oral antidiabetic agents to prevent the disease and maintain good metabolic control over the long term has motivated research on new physiological pathways involved in glucose homeostasis. The use of agents based on the effect of incretin hormones for the treatment of T2DM is quite promising. These treatments act through a mechanism that is distinct from that of drugs that have been commonly used in the treatment of this pathology. Furthermore, these agents reduce blood glucose levels to a level similar to other oral hypoglycemic agents with a minimal risk of hypoglycemia, they have few side effects, and they have no immediate need for dose titration.

However, although some of these agents have already been approved for the treatment of type 2 diabetes by regulatory authorities, phase IV studies and clinical experience are necessary to establish their actual benefits with greater certainty. The extra-glycemic effects, safety profiles and advantages and disadvantages compared to classically used oral antidiabetics remain to be fully characterized.

The increasing availability of numerous classes of medications has given clinicians and patients more therapeutic choices and perhaps an improved ability to achieve glycemic goals.

Author details

Roberto Pontarolo[1*], Andréia Cristina Conegero Sanches[2], Astrid Wiens[1],
Helena Hiemisch Lobo Borba[1], Luana Lenzi[1] and Suelem Tavares da Silva Penteado[1]

*Address all correspondence to: pontarolo@ufpr.br

1 Department of Pharmacy – Federal University of Paraná, Curitiba, Paraná, Brazil

2 Department of Medical and Pharmaceutical Sciences - State University of West of Paraná, Cascavel, Paraná, Brazil

References

[1] World Health Organization. http://www.who.int/en/. (acessed 5 november 2012).

[2] George PM, Valabhji J, Dawood M, Henry JA. Screening for Type 2 diabetes in the accident and emergency department. Diabet Med 2005;22(12):1766-9.

[3] Chopra M, Galbraith S, Darnton-Hill I. A global response to a global problem: the epidemic of overnutrition. Bull World Health Organ 2002;80(12):952-8.

[4] Zimmet P, Shaw J, Alberti KG. Preventing Type 2 diabetes and the dysmetabolic syndrome in the real world: a realistic view. Diabet Med 2003;20(9):693-702.

[5]   U.S. Department of Health and Human Services. NDIC: National Diabetes Statistics. http://diabetesniddknihgov/dm/pubs/statistics/#fast 2011. acessed in 12 november 2012.

[6]   Boog M, Magrini V. Relato de experiência: reeducação alimentar por meio de aborda-gem interdisciplinar envolvendo as áreas de Nutrição e Saúde Mental. Revista da So-ciedade de Cardiologia do Estado de São Paulo 1999;9(3):1-8.

[7]   Hirsch I, Riddle M. Current therapies for diabetes. Endocr Clin North Am 1997 1997;26:3.

[8]   Pan XR, Li GW, Hu YH, Wang JX, Yang WY, An ZX, et al. Effects of diet and exercise in preventing NIDDM in people with impaired glucose tolerance. The Da Qing IGT and Diabetes Study. Diabetes Care 1997;20(4):537-44.

[9]   Hepler CD, Strand LM. Opportunities and responsibilities in pharmaceutical care. Am J Hosp Pharm 1990;47(3):533-43.

[10] American Diabetes Association. Economic consequences of diabetes mellitus in the U.S. in 1997. American Diabetes Association. Diabetes Care 1998;21(2):296-309.

[11] Donovan JL, Blake DR. Patient non-compliance: deviance or reasoned decision-mak-ing? Soc Sci Med 1992;34(5):507-13.

[12] Association AD. Standards of medical care in diabetes--2008. Diabetes Care 2008;31 Suppl 1:S12-54.

[13] Farmaco AId. L'uso dei farmaci in Italia - Rapporto nazionale anno 2007. 2007.

[14] Anderson J. Obesity. Br Med J 1972;1(5799):560-3.

[15] Cusi K, DeFronzo R. Metformin: a review of its metabolic effects. Diabetes Rev 1998;6:89-131.

[16] Santos RF, Nomizo R, Wajhenberg BL, Reaven GM, Azhar S. Changes in insulin re-ceptor tyrosine kinase activity associated with metformin treatment of type 2 diabe-tes. Diabete Metab 1995;21(4):274-80.

[17] Johansen K. Efficacy of metformin in the treatment of NIDDM. Meta-analysis. Diabe-tes Care 1999;22(1):33-7.

[18] Araújo L, Britto MdS, Cruz T. Tratamento do Diabetes Mellitns do Tipo 2: Novas Op-ções. Arq Bras Endocrinol Metab 2000;44(6):509-18.

[19] Group U. Effect of intensive blood-glucose control with metformin on complications in overweight patients with type 2 diabetes (UKPDS 34). UK Prospective Diabetes Study (UKPDS) Group. Lancet 1998;352(9131):854-65.

[20] Chiasson JL, Josse RG, Hunt JA, Palmason C, Rodger NW, Ross SA, et al. The efficacy of acarbose in the treatment of patients with non-insulin-dependent diabetes melli-tus. A multicenter controlled clinical trial. Ann Intern Med 1994;121(12):928-35.

[21] DeFronzo R, Goodman A. The multicenter metformin study group: efficacy of metformin in NIDDM patients poorly controlled on diet done or diet plus sulfonylurea. N Engl J Med 1995;333:541-9.

[22] Inzucchi SE, Maggs DG, Spollett GR, Page SL, Rife FS, Walton V, et al. Efficacy and metabolic effects of metformin and troglitazone in type II diabetes mellitus. N Engl J Med 1998;338(13):867-72.

[23] Moses R, Slobodniuk R, Boyages S, Colagiuri S, Kidson W, Carter J, et al. Effect of repaglinide addition to metformin monotherapy on glycemic control in patients with type 2 diabetes. Diabetes Care 1999;22(1):119-24.

[24] Hirsch IB. Metformin added to insulin therapy in poorly controlled type 2 diabetes. Diabetes Care 1999;22(5):854.

[25] Turban S, Stretton C, Drouin O, Green CJ, Watson ML, Gray A, et al. Defining the contribution of AMP-activated protein kinase (AMPK) and protein kinase C (PKC) in regulation of glucose uptake by metformin in skeletal muscle cells. J Biol Chem 2012;287(24):20088-99.

[26] Flier JS. Diabetes. The missing link with obesity? Nature 2001;409(6818):292-3.

[27] Kahn SE, Haffner SM, Heise MA, Herman WH, Holman RR, Jones NP, et al. Glycemic durability of rosiglitazone, metformin, or glyburide monotherapy. N Engl J Med 2006;355(23):2427-43.

[28] Olokoba AB, Obateru OA, Olokoba LB. Type 2 diabetes mellitus: a review of current trends. Oman Med J 2012;27(4):269-73.

[29] Silva A, Lazaretti-Castro M. Diabetes melito, tiazolidinedionas e fraturas: uma história inacabada. Arq Bras Endocrinol Metab 2010;54(4):345-51.

[30] Horton ES, Whitehouse F, Ghazzi MN, Venable TC, Whitcomb RW. Troglitazone in combination with sulfonylurea restores glycemic control in patients with type 2 diabetes. The Troglitazone Study Group. Diabetes Care 1998;21(9):1462-9.

[31] Iwamoto Y, Kosaka K, Kuzuya T, Akanuma Y, Shigeta Y, Kaneko T. Effect of combination therapy of troglitazone and sulphonylureas in patients with Type 2 diabetes who were poorly controlled by sulphonylurea therapy alone. Diabet Med 1996;13(4): 365-70.

[32] Day C. Thiazolidinediones: a new class of antidiabetic drugs. Diabet Med 1999;16(3): 179-92.

[33] Balfour JA, Plosker GL. Rosiglitazone. Drugs 1999;57(6):921-30; discussion 31-2.

[34] Grey A. Skeletal consequences of thiazolidinedione therapy. Osteoporos Int 2008;19(2):129-37.

[35] van de Laar FA. Alpha-glucosidase inhibitors in the early treatment of type 2 diabe-
      tes. Vasc Health Risk Manag 2008;4(6):1189-95.

[36] Inzucchi SE, Bergenstal RM, Buse JB, Diamant M, Ferrannini E, Nauck M, et al. Man-
      agement of hyperglycemia in type 2 diabetes: a patient-centered approach: position
      statement of the American Diabetes Association (ADA) and the European Associa-
      tion for the Study of Diabetes (EASD). Diabetes Care 2012;35(6):1364-79.

[37] Rosak C, Mertes G. Critical evaluation of the role of acarbose in the treatment of dia-
      betes: patient considerations. Diabetes Metab Syndr Obes 2012;5:357-67.

[38] Coniff R, Krol A. Acarbose: a review of US clinical experience. Clin Ther 1997;19(1):
      16-26; discussion 2-3.

[39] Lebovitz HE. alpha-Glucosidase inhibitors. Endocrinol Metab Clin North Am
      1997;26(3):539-51.

[40] Braun D, Schönherr U, Mitzkat H. Efficacy of acarbose monotherapy in patients with
      type 2 diabetes: a double-blind study conducted in general practice. Endocrinol Me-
      tabol 1996;3:275-80.

[41] Coniff RF, Shapiro JA, Seaton TB, Hoogwerf BJ, Hunt JA. A double-blind placebo-
      controlled trial evaluating the safety and efficacy of acarbose for the treatment of pa-
      tients with insulin-requiring type II diabetes. Diabetes Care 1995;18(7):928-32.

[42] van de Laar FA, Lucassen PL, Akkermans RP, van de Lisdonk EH, Rutten GE, van
      Weel C. Alpha-glucosidase inhibitors for patients with type 2 diabetes: results from a
      Cochrane systematic review and meta-analysis. Diabetes Care 2005;28(1):154-63.

[43] Holman RR. Long-term efficacy of sulfonylureas: a United Kingdom Prospective
      Diabetes Study perspective. Metabolism 2006;55(5 Suppl 1):S2-5.

[44] Wannmacher L. Antidiabéticos orais: comparação entre diferentes intervenções. Uso
      Racional de medicamentos: temas relacionados - Organização Pan-Americana da
      Saúde/Organização Mundial da Saúde 2005;2(11).

[45] Rang H, Dale M, Ritter J. Farmacologia. 4 ed. Rio de Janeiro: Guanabara Koogan;
      2001.

[46] Akalin S, Berntorp K, Ceriello A, Das AK, Kilpatrick ES, Koblik T, et al. Intensive glu-
      cose therapy and clinical implications of recent data: a consensus statement from the
      Global Task Force on Glycaemic Control. Int J Clin Pract 2009;63(10):1421-5.

[47] Lee SJ, Eng C. Goals of glycemic control in frail older patients with diabetes. Jama
      2011;305(13):1350-1.

[48] Basit A, Riaz M, Fawwad A. Glimepiride: evidence-based facts, trends, and observa-
      tions. Vasc Health Risk Manag 2012;8:463-72.

[49] Holstein A, Plaschke A, Egberts EH. Lower incidence of severe hypoglycaemia in patients with type 2 diabetes treated with glimepiride versus glibenclamide. Diabetes Metab Res Rev 2001;17(6):467-73.

[50] Gangji AS, Cukierman T, Gerstein HC, Goldsmith CH, Clase CM. A systematic review and meta-analysis of hypoglycemia and cardiovascular events: a comparison of glyburide with other secretagogues and with insulin. Diabetes Care 2007;30(2): 389-94.

[51] Ben-Ami H, Nagachandran P, Mendelson A, Edoute Y. Drug-induced hypoglycemic coma in 102 diabetic patients. Arch Intern Med 1999;159(3):281-4.

[52] Ferner RE, Neil HA. Sulphonylureas and hypoglycaemia. Br Med J (Clin Res Ed) 1988;296(6627):949-50.

[53] Shorr RI, Ray WA, Daugherty JR, Griffin MR. Individual sulfonylureas and serious hypoglycemia in older people. J Am Geriatr Soc 1996;44(7):751-5.

[54] Bugos C, Austin M, Atherton T, Viereck C. Long-term treatment of type 2 diabetes mellitus with glimepiride is weight neutral: a meta-analysis. Diabetes Res Clin Pract 2000;50(1):S47.

[55] Martin S, Kolb H, Beuth J, van Leendert R, Schneider B, Scherbaum WA. Change in patients' body weight after 12 months of treatment with glimepiride or glibenclamide in Type 2 diabetes: a multicentre retrospective cohort study. Diabetologia 2003;46(12):1611-7.

[56] Lazdunski M. Ion channel effects of antidiabetic sulfonylureas. Horm Metab Res 1996;28(9):488-95.

[57] Rosenstock J, Hassman DR, Madder RD, Brazinsky SA, Farrell J, Khutoryansky N, et al. Repaglinide versus nateglinide monotherapy: a randomized, multicenter study. Diabetes Care 2004;27(6):1265-70.

[58] Derosa G, Mugellini A, Ciccarelli L, Crescenzi G, Fogari R. Comparison between repaglinide and glimepiride in patients with type 2 diabetes mellitus: a one-year, randomized, double-blind assessment of metabolic parameters and cardiovascular risk factors. Clin Ther 2003;25(2):472-84.

[59] Stephens JW, Bodvarsdottir TB, Wareham K, Prior SL, Bracken RM, Lowe GD, et al. Effects of short-term therapy with glibenclamide and repaglinide on incretin hormones and oxidative damage associated with postprandial hyperglycaemia in people with type 2 diabetes mellitus. Diabetes Res Clin Pract 2011;94(2):199-206.

[60] Reimann F, Proks P, Ashcroft FM. Effects of mitiglinide (S 21403) on Kir6.2/SUR1, Kir6.2/SUR2A and Kir6.2/SUR2B types of ATP-sensitive potassium channel. Br J Pharmacol 2001;132(7):1542-8.

[61] Wolffenbuttel BH, Nijst L, Sels JP, Menheere PP, Muller PG, Kruseman AC. Effects of a new oral hypoglycaemic agent, repaglinide, on metabolic control in sulphonylurea-treated patients with NIDDM. Eur J Clin Pharmacol 1993;45(2):113-6.

[62] Dornhorst A. Insulinotropic meglitinide analogues. Lancet 2001;358(9294):1709-16.

[63] Papa G, Fedele V, Rizzo MR, Fioravanti M, Leotta C, Solerte SB, et al. Safety of type 2 diabetes treatment with repaglinide compared with glibenclamide in elderly people: A randomized, open-label, two-period, cross-over trial. Diabetes Care 2006;29(8): 1918-20.

[64] Keilson L, Mather S, Walter YH, Subramanian S, McLeod JF. Synergistic effects of nateglinide and meal administration on insulin secretion in patients with type 2 diabetes mellitus. J Clin Endocrinol Metab 2000;85(3):1081-6.

[65] Tentolouris N, Voulgari C, Katsilambros N. A review of nateglinide in the management of patients with type 2 diabetes. Vasc Health Risk Manag 2007;3(6):797-807.

[66] Fehse F, Trautmann M, Holst JJ, Halseth AE, Nanayakkara N, Nielsen LL, et al. Exenatide augments first- and second-phase insulin secretion in response to intravenous glucose in subjects with type 2 diabetes. J Clin Endocrinol Metab 2005;90(11):5991-7.

[67] Brown DX, Evans M. Choosing between GLP-1 Receptor Agonists and DPP-4 Inhibitors: A Pharmacological Perspective. J Nutr Metab 2012;2012:381713.

[68] Holst JJ, Deacon CF, Vilsboll T, Krarup T, Madsbad S. Glucagon-like peptide-1, glucose homeostasis and diabetes. Trends Mol Med 2008;14(4):161-8.

[69] Buse JB, Rosenstock J, Sesti G, Schmidt WE, Montanya E, Brett JH, et al. Liraglutide once a day versus exenatide twice a day for type 2 diabetes: a 26-week randomised, parallel-group, multinational, open-label trial (LEAD-6). Lancet 2009;374(9683):39-47.

[70] Kendall DM, Riddle MC, Rosenstock J, Zhuang D, Kim DD, Fineman MS, et al. Effects of exenatide (exendin-4) on glycemic control over 30 weeks in patients with type 2 diabetes treated with metformin and a sulfonylurea. Diabetes Care 2005;28(5): 1083-91.

[71] Iltz JL, Baker DE, Setter SM, Keith Campbell R. Exenatide: an incretin mimetic for the treatment of type 2 diabetes mellitus. Clin Ther 2006;28(5):652-65.

[72] Inoue K, Maeda N, Kashine S, Fujishima Y, Kozawa J, Hiuge-Shimizu A, et al. Short-term effects of liraglutide on visceral fat adiposity, appetite, and food preference: a pilot study of obese Japanese patients with type 2 diabetes. Cardiovasc Diabetol 2012;10:109.

[73] Bloomgarden Z, Drexler A. What role will 'gliptins' play in glycemic control? Cleve Clin J Med 2008;75(4):305-10.

[74] Zerilli T, Pyon EY. Sitagliptin phosphate: a DPP-4 inhibitor for the treatment of type 2 diabetes mellitus. Clin Ther 2007;29(12):2614-34.

[75] Gallwitz B. Review of sitagliptin phosphate: a novel treatment for type 2 diabetes. Vasc Health Risk Manag 2007;3(2):203-10.

[76] Nathan DM. Finding new treatments for diabetes--how many, how fast.. how good? N Engl J Med 2007;356(5):437-40.

[77] Ye Z, Chen L, Yang Z, Li Q, Huang Y, He M, et al. Metabolic effects of fluoxetine in adults with type 2 diabetes mellitus: a meta-analysis of randomized placebo-controlled trials. PLoS One 2011;6(7):e21551.

[78] Mancini MC, Halpern A. Pharmacological treatment of obesity. Arq Bras Endocrinol Metabol 2006;50(2):377-89.

[79] Fuchs F, Wannmacher L, Ferreira M. Farmacologia clínica: fundamentos da terapêutica racional. Rio de Janeiro: Guanabara Koogan; 2004.

[80] Ioannides-Demos LL, Piccenna L, McNeil JJ. Pharmacotherapies for obesity: past, current, and future therapies. J Obes 2011;2011:179674.

[81] Kang JG, Park CY. Anti-Obesity Drugs: A Review about Their Effects and Safety. Diabetes Metab J 2012;36(1):13-25.

[82] Heal DJ, Gosden J, Smith SL. Regulatory challenges for new drugs to treat obesity and comorbid metabolic disorders. Br J Clin Pharmacol 2009;68(6):861-74.

[83] Sargent BJ, Moore NA. New central targets for the treatment of obesity. Br J Clin Pharmacol 2009;68(6):852-60.

[84] Li M, Cheung BM. Pharmacotherapy for obesity. Br J Clin Pharmacol 2009;68(6): 804-10.

[85] Maia F, Melo F. Substituição da insulina NPH por insulina glargina em uma coorte de pacientes diabéticos: estudo observacional. Arquivos Brasileiros de Endocrinologia & Metabologia 2007;51(3):426-30.

[86] Pires A, Chacra A. A evolução da insulinoterapia no diabetes melito tipo 1. Endocrinol Metab 2008;52(2):268-78.

[87] Wajchenberg B, Forti A, Ferreira S, Oliveira O, Lopes C, Lerário A, et al. Menor incidência de hipoglicemia noturna com o uso de insulina lispro comparada à insulina humana regular no tratamento de pacientes com diabetes do tipo 1. Arq Bras Endocrinol Metab 2000;44(2):133-8.

[88] Home PD, Rosskamp R, Forjanic-Klapproth J, Dressler A. A randomized multicentre trial of insulin glargine compared with NPH insulin in people with type 1 diabetes. Diabetes Metab Res Rev 2005;21(6):545-53.

[89] Kurtzhals P. Pharmacology of insulin detemir. Endocrinol Metab Clin North Am 2007;36 Suppl 1:14-20.

[90] Soran H, Younis N. Insulin detemir: a new basal insulin analogue. Diabetes Obes Metab 2006;8(1):26-30.

[91] Rollin G, Punales N. Utilização da insulina glargina em crianças menores de oito anos de idade. Arq Bras Endocrinol Metab 2009;53(6):721-25.

[92] Vazquez-Carrera M, Silvestre JS. Insulin analogues in the management of diabetes. Methods Find Exp Clin Pharmacol 2004;26(6):445-61.

[93] Bailey CJ, Barnett AH. Inhaled insulin: new formulation, new trial. Lancet 2010;375(9733):2199-201.

[94] Siekmeier R, Scheuch G. Inhaled insulin--does it become reality? J Physiol Pharmacol 2008;59 Suppl 6:81-113.

[95] Mastrandrea LD. Inhaled insulin: overview of a novel route of insulin administration. Vasc Health Risk Manag 2010;6:47-58.

[96] Arnolds S, Heise T. Inhaled insulin. Best Pract Res Clin Endocrinol Metab 2007;21(4): 555-71.

[97] Tibaldi JM. Evolution of insulin development: focus on key parameters. Adv Ther 2012;29(7):590-619.

[98] Carvalheira J, Saad M. Insulin resistance/hyperinsulinemia associated diseases not included in the metabolic syndrome. Arq bras endocrinol metab 2006;50(2):360-7.

[99] Janghorbani M, Dehghani M, Salehi-Marzijarani M. Systematic review and meta-analysis of insulin therapy and risk of cancer. Horm Cancer 2012;3(4):137-46.

Chapter 6

Insulin Therapy for Diabetes

Shara S. Azad, Esma R. Isenovic,
Subhashini Yaturu and Shaker A. Mousa

Additional information is available at the end of the chapter

1. Introduction

Diabetes affects 25.8 million people, or 8.3% of the U.S. population. Among people with diabetes, 26% are insulin users.[1] Therapy with insulin is effective at lowering blood glucose in patients with diabetes. Insulin is a key player in the control of diabetes for patients with type 1, and it is required at later stages by patients with type 2. Hyperglycemia in type 1 diabetes is a result of the deficiency of insulin, and in type 2 diabetes hyperglycemia is due to impaired tissue response to insulin.

The discovery of insulin is hailed as one of the most dramatic events in the history of the treatment of disease. It was isolated in 1921, with its first clinical use in 1922.[2] The major advances achieved in this area include the human insulin analogue synthesis. Insulin delivery systems currently available for insulin administration include syringes, infusion pumps, jet injectors, and pens. The traditional and most predictable method for insulin administration is by subcutaneous injections. The major drawback of current forms of insulin therapy is their invasive nature. In type 1 diabetes, good glycemic control usually requires at least two, three, or more daily insulin injections. To decrease the suffering, the use of supersonic injectors, infusion pumps, sharp needles, and pens has been adopted.

Such invasive and intensive techniques have spurred the search for alternative, more pleasant methods for administering insulin. Several non-invasive approaches for insulin delivery are being pursued. The ultimate goal is to eliminate the need to deliver insulin exogenously and for patients to regain the ability to produce and use their own insulin. The success of the administration route is measured by its ability to elicit effective and predictable lowering of blood glucose level, therefore minimizing the risk of diabetic complications. Newer methods explored include the artificial pancreas with a closed-loop system, transdermal insulin, and buccal, oral, pulmonary, nasal, ocular, and rectal routes. This chapter focuses on the new methods that are being explored for use in the future.

2. Current methods in insulin therapy

Current methods of insulin delivery include using syringes, continuous subcutaneous insulin infusion (CSII), and insulin pens. Use of syringes is the most common method, and there is a wide choice of products that are easy to read and operate. CSII, also referred to as an insulin pump system, is designed to provide a continuous supply of insulin infusion around the clock and can be individualized and adjusted as per the specific needs of the patient. CSII is a way to simulate the physiology of daily insulin secretion where an appropriate level of insulin is delivered. The use of an insulin pump is superior to multi-dose insulin injections because it is easier to use and therefore provides the patient with more flexibility. A disadvantage is that insulin pump therapy is expensive compared to the use of traditional syringes and vials.

Insulin pen devices offer an alternative method for insulin delivery that is more accurate and less painful versus vials and syringes.[3] Reusable insulin pens offer a number of advantages including durability and flexibility in carrying a multiple days' supply.

3. Future trends (Table 1)

Injectable insulin: Two promising new insulin preparations include a long-acting basal insulin analogue called insulin degludec and an ultrafast-acting insulin analogue, human insulin Linjeta™ (formally called VIAject®).

Insulin degludec is novel, ultra-long-acting basal insulin.[4] Insulin degludec is almost identical to human insulin in structure except for the last amino acid deleted from the B-chain and addition of a glutamyl link from LysB29 to a hexadecandioic fatty acid.[4] It forms soluble multi-hexamers after subcutaneous injection, resulting in an ultra-long action profile with a half life of more than 24 hours.

Insulin degludec has proven to be non-inferior to currently available, long-acting insulin analogue insulin glargine in trials carried out in both type 1 and type 2 diabetes.[5-6] In an exploratory phase 2 trial in subjects with type 1 diabetes, insulin degludec was found to be safe and well tolerated and had comparable glycemic control to insulin glargine, but with reduced rates of hypoglycemia.[7] In a multicenter phase 3 clinical trial in adults with type 1 diabetes, at one year, compared to insulin glargine, glycemic control was similar to glycemic control using glargine with decreased nocturnal hypoglycemia.[6] Similarly, in an open-label phase 3 non-inferiority trial in type 2 diabetes patients, improvement in glycemic control was comparable to insulin glargine at one year follow-up (drop in HbA1C by 1.1% in the degludec group and 1.2% in the glargine group) with fewer hypoglycemic episodes in insulin degludec users.[5] Insulin degludec is not yet approved by the FDA.

Linjeta™, formally called VIAject®, is recombinant human insulin with a fast onset of action. In a study of pharmacodynamics and pharmacokinetic properties of an ultrafast insulin, it was found to have an earlier onset of action and shorter time to maximal plasma insulin concentration. VIAject®, compared to human insulin, had less within-subject variability of plasma insulin.[8] In a double blind, three-way crossover study with VIAject® compared to lispro insulin, VIAject® was found to be bioequivalent to the previously used formulation and had a faster absorption/onset of action than insulin lispro.[9] VIAject® is currently undergoing two pivotal phase 3 clinical studies for both type 1 and type 2 diabetes. Since the VIAject® pharmacodynamics mimic 1st phase release insulin and the amount of insulin circulating several hours after a meal, it leads to possible reduction in hypoglycemia, and it is predicted to possibly prevent weight gain.[8]

Artificial pancreas: Closed-loop insulin delivery is an emerging therapeutic approach for people with type 1 diabetes. [10] Even with the use of continuous glucose monitors and insulin pumps, most people with type 1 diabetes do not achieve glycemic goals and continue to have unacceptable rates of hypoglycemia. The goal of closed-loop therapy is to achieve good glycemic control with the use of a control algorithm that directs insulin delivery according to glucose levels while reducing the risk of hypoglycemia. Insulin delivery in the closed-loop system is modulated at intervals of 1-15 minutes, depending on interstitial glucose levels. The uniqueness of this approach is the real-time response of insulin delivery to the glucose levels, similar to that of the beta-cell. The algorithms that are most relevant include the proportional-integral-derivative control (PID) and the model-predictive control (MPC).[11]

Several areas need improvement to have a near normal closed-loop system. First and foremost is the rapid onset of action. The lag period of current fast-acting insulin analogs is 90-120 minutes. Current trials show promise. In a phase 2 study with or without recombinant human hyaluronidase (rHuPH20) that accelerates insulin absorption in healthy volunteers, both lispro and recombinant human insulin with rHuPH20 produced earlier and greater peak insulin concentrations, improved postprandial glycemic control, and reduced hypoglycemia.[12]

Rapid acting insulins are being developed that use monomeric insulins that cannot form hexamers.[13] As mentioned earlier, ultrafast insulin VIAject®, a formulation of human soluble insulin, improves the rate of insulin absorption. It has been reported in a study to evaluate its pharmacodynamics and pharmacokinetic properties that VIAject® has higher metabolic activity in the first two hours after injection [14] True closed-loop systems, which determine minute-to-minute insulin delivery based on continuous glucose sensor data in real time, have shown promise in small inpatient feasibility studies using a variety of algorithmic and hormonal approaches.

Buccal delivery of insulin: The buccal delivery system for insulin delivers insulin through an aerosol spray into the oral cavity and hence differs from inhalers. The insulin is absorbed through the inside of the cheeks and in the back of the mouth instead of the lungs. In vivo studies performed on diabetic rats showed promising results with stable blood glucose profile with a significant hypoglycemic response after 7 hours using buccal insulin.[15] Similar studies in the rabbit and rat have shown that buccal spray of insulin is an effective insulin delivery system, which is promising for clinical trial and future clinical application.[16] Though promising in rat models, they are not appropriate models because rats have a keratinized buccal mucosa. The only animal models with comparable human buccal permeability are pigs.

Oral-lynTM: Generex Biotechnology Corporation (Toronto, Canada) is developing a buccal insulin formulation based on RapidMistTM, an advanced buccal drug delivery technology. [17] Oral-lynTM is a liquid formulation of human regular insulin with a spray propellant for prandial insulin therapy. The formulation results in an aerosol with relatively large micelles where the majority of the particles have a mean size >10 µm and therefore cannot go into the lungs. Each puff is claimed to deliver 10 U of insulin. The absorption rate of administered insulin as a puff is 10%, and that corresponds to 1 U when 1 puff of 10 U is delivered, which means 10 puffs will deliver 10 U insulin for a meal.[17]

Clinical studies in healthy volunteers and subjects with type 1 and type 2 diabetes have shown that the oral insulin spray was absorbed in direct relation to the amount given, and it had a rapid onset and a shorter duration compared with regular insulin given subcutaneously. In all of the studies conducted, the oral insulin spray was generally well tolerated. The only side effects included mild episodes of transient dizziness in some healthy volunteers and subjects with type 1 diabetes.[18] The product is on the market in a number of countries (e.g., Ecuador and India).[17] Without appropriately designed and performed phase 3 trials at hand, it is not possible to make any clear statement about the benefits/risk ratio of the different buccal insulins.[17]

Oral insulin: Oral insulin has benefits in terms of compliance among patients, as well as physiological advantages because oral insulin can mimic the physiological fate of insulin through first pass to the liver, directly and effectively inhibiting hepatic glucose production. [19] Since the initial discovery of insulin by Banting and Best in 1922, the oral form of insulin has been the elusive goal. Difficulties encountered for oral insulin delivery, since it is a protein, include degradation by the low pH of the stomach and the digestive enzymes in the stomach and small intestine. The major barrier for insulin absorption is the intestinal epithelium. All these factors lead to low bioavailability, and that leads to significant inter- and intra-subject variability.

Nanotechnologies have brought some hope for improved delivery of insulin. Nanotechnology applications for delivery of hydrophilic drugs such as insulin might be achieved using biodegradable polymers such as chitosan, which has been extensively exploited for the preparation of nanoparticles for oral controlled delivery of several therapeutic agents.[20-24] In recent years, chitosan cross-linked to various hydrophobic polymers has been utilized for the preparation of orally delivered drugs because of improved permeation and sustained release characteristics.[25-26]

The newer products that are being tried include water-soluble, long-acting insulin derivative, [(2-sulfo)-9-fluorenylmethoxycarbonyl]3-insulin,[27] vitamin B12-dextran nano particles,[28] lipid nanoparticles,[29] and PEGylated calcium phosphate nanoparticles as oral carriers for insulin.[30] Protection of insulin from the gastric environment has been achieved by coating the nanoparticles with a pH-sensitive polymer that dissolves in the intestine at mild alkaline pH. In rats, oral insulin nanoformulation significantly (*P*<0.05) reduced blood glucose in normal and diabetic rats.[31]

Biocon (Bangalore, India) is manufacturing IN-105, which is in late phase 3.[17] IN-105 is a human recombinant insulin conjugated with polyethylene glycol via an acetyl chain. It is orally bioavailable and stable at ambient conditions. Preclinical studies in different species have shown acceptable efficacy and safety. Its maximal circulating insulin levels after oral administration of 5 mg were observed after 20 minutes, and the maximum drop in glucose occurred at 40 minutes after oral administration. Phase 1 and phase 2 trials demonstrated that the absorption of IN-105 and the reduction in blood glucose levels were proportional to the dose administered.[32]

Inhaled insulin: The inhaled products fall into two main groups: the dry powder formulations and solution, which are delivered through different inhaler systems. Exubera®, containing rapid-acting insulin in powder form, was studied in patients with type 1 and type 2 diabetes mellitus.[33-34] The results of a patient preference study, using a comparison of utility scores, showed a greater preference for the inhaled route over insulin injection.[35] However, issues like cost, the bulkiness of the device, and the small number of studies in subjects with underlying respiratory disease prevented widespread use of this new mode of delivery.[36-37] Exubera® was available for less than one year, and then Pfizer took it off the market in 2007 because the drug failed to gain market acceptance.

Afrezza®: (MannKind Corporation, Valencia, CA, USA) is recombinant human insulin, using the Technosphere® concept and administered using a next-generation inhaler called Dreamboat®. Technosphere® is a drug delivery system created by micro particles (2-3 μm) that form microspheres, which are then lyophilized into a dry powder for inhalation.[38]

Transdermal insulin: Transdermal insulin delivery is a needle-free alternative and avoids the disadvantages associated with other alternative routes such as the pulmonary and nasal routes. Permeation of compounds is limited to small, lipophilic molecules. The stratum corneum, the outermost layer of the skin, constitutes the major barrier for insulin permeation to reach useful levels. Several chemical and physical enhancement techniques such as iontophoresis, ultrasound/sonophoresis, micro-needles, electroporation, laser ablation, and chemical enhancers have been explored to overcome the stratum corneum barrier to increase skin permeability.

Methods to improve transdermal delivery:

1. Chemical enhancers, which alter the lipid structure of the stratum.

2. Iontophoresis, which enhances the transdermal delivery of compounds via the use of a small electric current.[39]

3. Micro-needle technology, which involves the creation of micron-sized channels in the skin, thereby disrupting the stratum corneum barrier[40] and delivering the drug into the epidermis without disruption of nerve endings.[41]

4. Sonophoresis, which uses ultrasound and has been shown to increase skin permeability of insulin. It is still being evaluated.[42]

4. Conclusions

Effective glycemic control remains an important clinical goal. Patient barriers to accepting insulin initiation include fear of hypoglycemia, weight gain, and the inflexible timing of scheduled insulin doses, leading to adherence issues. Additionally, the invasive nature of the insulin syringe, pump, and pen remains an obstacle for patients. Of the alternatives to subcutaneous and injected insulin, intranasal, inhalable, and oral insulin could prove to be the most cost-effective ones. Oral insulin in particular could prove to be promising, especially since as a therapy it seems to have progressed with nanotechnology research, allowing for several types of encapsulations to bypass the gastric acidic environment. Artificial pancreas or closing the loop with insulin pumps that deliver insulin in response to sensors also appears to be promising.

Method	Mechanism
Artificial pancreas	Insulin pump controlled by algorithm with glucose monitor
Buccal insulin	Insulin through an aerosol spray
Oral insulin	Various nanoparticle encasings bound to insulin
Inhalable insulin	Insulin absorbed through alveolar membranes
Transdermal insulin (patches)	Insulin absorbed through pores in skin opened with ultrasound energy, microdermabrasion, etc.
Intranasal insulin	Absorbed through nasal mucosae

Table 1. Methods for Future Types of Insulin Therapy

Author details

Shara S. Azad[1], Esma R. Isenovic[2], Subhashini Yaturu[3] and Shaker A. Mousa[1*]

*Address all correspondence to: Shaker.Mousa@acphs.edu

1 Pharmaceutical Research Institute, Albany College of Pharmacy and Health Sciences, 1 Discovery Drive, Rensselaer, NY, USA

2 Vinca Institute, University of Belgrade, Department for Molecular Genetics and Radiobiology, Belgrade, Serbia

3 Stratton Veterans Affairs Medical Center /Albany Medical College, Albany, NY, USA

References

[1] National Diabetes Statistics, 2011. U.S. Department of Health and Human Services; 2011. http://diabetes.niddk.nih.gov/dm/pubs/statistics/#fast. Accessed 15 November, 2012.

[2] Rosenfeld L. Insulin: discovery and controversy. Clin Chem. 2002;48(12) 2270-88.

[3] Magwire ML. Addressing barriers to insulin therapy: the role of insulin pens. Am J Ther. 2011;18(5) 392-402.

[4] Danne T, Bolinder J. New insulins and insulin therapy. Int J Clin Pract Suppl. 2011;65(Suppl 170) 26-30.

[5] Garber AJ, King AB, Del Prato S, Sreenan S, Balci MK, Munoz-Torres M, et al. Insulin degludec, an ultra-longacting basal insulin, versus insulin glargine in basal-bolus treatment with mealtime insulin aspart in type 2 diabetes (BEGIN Basal-Bolus Type 2): a phase 3, randomised, open-label, treat-to-target non-inferiority trial. Lancet. 2012;379(9825) 1498-507.

[6] Heller S, Buse J, Fisher M, Garg S, Marre M, Merker L, et al. Insulin degludec, an ultra-longacting basal insulin, versus insulin glargine in basal-bolus treatment with mealtime insulin aspart in type 1 diabetes (BEGIN Basal-Bolus Type 1): a phase 3, randomised, open-label, treat-to-target non-inferiority trial. Lancet. 2012;379(9825) 1489-97.

[7] Birkeland KI, Home PD, Wendisch U, Ratner RE, Johansen T, Endahl LA, et al. Insulin degludec in type 1 diabetes: a randomized controlled trial of a new-generation ultra-long-acting insulin compared with insulin glargine. Diabetes Care. 2011;34(3) 661-5.

[8] Hompesch M, McManus L, Pohl R, Simms P, Pfutzner A, Bulow E, et al. Intra-individual variability of the metabolic effect of a novel rapid-acting insulin (VIAject) in comparison to regular human insulin. J Diabetes Sci Technol. 2008;2(4) 568-71.

[9] Heinemann L, Nosek L, Flacke F, Albus K, Krasner A, Pichotta P, et al. U-100, pH-Neutral formulation of VIAject(®) : faster onset of action than insulin lispro in patients with type 1 diabetes. Diabetes Obes Metab. 2012;14(3) 222-7.

[10] Elleri D, Dunger DB, Hovorka R. Closed-loop insulin delivery for treatment of type 1 diabetes. BMC Med. 2011;9 120.

[11] Radziuk J. The artificial pancreas. Diabetes. 2012;61(9) 2221-4.

[12] Hompesch M, Muchmore DB, Morrow L, Vaughn DE. Accelerated insulin pharmacokinetics and improved postprandial glycemic control in patients with type 1 diabetes after coadministration of prandial insulins with hyaluronidase. Diabetes Care. 2011;34(3) 666-8.

[13] Brange J, Owens DR, Kang S, Volund A. Monomeric insulins and their experimental and clinical implications. Diabetes Care. 1990;13(9) 923-54.

[14] Steiner S, Hompesch M, Pohl R, Simms P, Flacke F, Mohr T, et al. A novel insulin formulation with a more rapid onset of action. Diabetologia. 2008;51(9) 1602-6.

[15] Venugopalan P, Sapre A, Venkatesan N, Vyas SP. Pelleted bioadhesive polymeric nanoparticles for buccal delivery of insulin: preparation and characterization. Pharmazie. 2001;56(3) 217-9.

[16] Xu HB, Huang KX, Zhu YS, Gao QH, Wu QZ, Tian WQ, et al. Hypoglycaemic effect of a novel insulin buccal formulation on rabbits. Pharmacol Res. 2002;46(5) 459-67.

[17] Heinemann L, Jacques Y. Oral insulin and buccal insulin: a critical reappraisal. J Diabetes Sci Technol. 2009;3(3) 568-84.

[18] Pozzilli P, Raskin P, Parkin CG. Review of clinical trials: update on oral insulin spray formulation. Diabetes Obes Metab. 2010;12(2) 91-6.

[19] Arbit E, Kidron M. Oral insulin: the rationale for this approach and current developments. J Diabetes Sci Technol. 2009;3(3) 562-7.

[20] Trapani A, Lopedota A, Franco M, Cioffi N, Ieva E, Garcia-Fuentes M, et al. A comparative study of chitosan and chitosan/cyclodextrin nanoparticles as potential carriers for the oral delivery of small peptides. Eur J Pharm Biopharm. 2010;75(1) 26-32.

[21] Cui F, Qian F, Zhao Z, Yin L, Tang C, Yin C. Preparation, characterization, and oral delivery of insulin loaded carboxylated chitosan grafted poly(methyl methacrylate) nanoparticles. Biomacromolecules. 2009;10(5) 1253-8.

[22] Li T, Shi XW, Du YM, Tang YF. Quaternized chitosan/alginate nanoparticles for protein delivery. J Biomed Mater Res A. 2007;83(2) 383-90.

[23] Pan Y, Li YJ, Zhao HY, Zheng JM, Xu H, Wei G, et al. Bioadhesive polysaccharide in protein delivery system: chitosan nanoparticles improve the intestinal absorption of insulin in vivo. Int J Pharm. 2002;249(1-2) 139-47.

[24] Ma Z, Yeoh HH, Lim LY. Formulation pH modulates the interaction of insulin with chitosan nanoparticles. J Pharm Sci. 2002;91(6) 1396-404.

[25] Jose S, Fangueiro JF, Smitha J, Cinu TA, Chacko AJ, Premaletha K, et al. Cross-linked chitosan microspheres for oral delivery of insulin: Taguchi design and in vivo testing. Colloids Surf B Biointerfaces. 2012;92 175-9.

[26] Chaudhury A, Das S. Recent advancement of chitosan-based nanoparticles for oral controlled delivery of insulin and other therapeutic agents. AAPS PharmSciTech. 2011;12(1) 10-20.

[27] Sung HW, Sonaje K, Feng SS. Nanomedicine for diabetes treatment. Nanomedicine (Lond). 2011;6(8) 1297-300.

[28] Chalasani KB, Russell-Jones GJ, Jain AK, Diwan PV, Jain SK. Effective oral delivery of insulin in animal models using vitamin B12-coated dextran nanoparticles. J Control Release. 2007;122(2) 141-50.

[29] Severino P, Andreani T, Macedo AS, Fangueiro JF, Santana MH, Silva AM, et al. Current state-of-art and new trends on lipid nanoparticles (SLN and NLC) for oral drug delivery. J Drug Delivery. 2012;2012 750891.

[30] Ramachandran R, Paul W, Sharma CP. Synthesis and characterization of PEGylated calcium phosphate nanoparticles for oral insulin delivery. J Biomed Mater Res B Appl Biomater. 2009;88(1) 41-8.

[31] Najafzadeh H, Kooshapur H, Kianidehkordi F. Evaluation of an oral insulin formulation in normal and diabetic rats. Indian J Pharmacol. 2012;44(1) 103-5.

[32] Khedkar A, Iyer H, Anand A, Verma M, Krishnamurthy S, Savale S, et al. A dose range finding study of novel oral insulin (IN-105) under fed conditions in type 2 diabetes mellitus subjects. Diabetes Obes Metab. 2010;12(8) 659-64.

[33] Fineberg SE. Diabetes therapy trials with inhaled insulin. Expert Opin Investig Drugs. 2006;15(7) 743-62.

[34] Barnett AH. Exubera inhaled insulin: a review. Int J Clin Pract. 2004;58(4) 394-401.

[35] Chancellor J, Aballea S, Lawrence A, Sheldon R, Cure S, Plun-Favreau J, et al. Preferences of patients with diabetes mellitus for inhaled versus injectable insulin regimens. Pharmacoeconomics. 2008;26(3) 217-34.

[36] Zarogoulidis P, Papanas N, Kouliatsis G, Spyratos D, Zarogoulidis K, Maltezos E. Inhaled insulin: too soon to be forgotten? J Aerosol Med Pulm Drug Deliv. 2011;24(5) 213-23.

[37] Hegewald M, Crapo RO, Jensen RL. Pulmonary function changes related to acute and chronic administration of inhaled insulin. Diabetes Technol Ther. 2007;9 Suppl 1 S93-S101.

[38] Steiner S, Pfutzner A, Wilson BR, Harzer O, Heinemann L, Rave K. Technosphere/Insulin--proof of concept study with a new insulin formulation for pulmonary delivery. Exp Clin Endocrinol Diabetes. 2002;110(1) 17-21.

[39] Batheja P, Thakur R, Michniak B. Transdermal iontophoresis. Expert Opin Drug Deliv. 2006;3(1) 127-38.

[40] Chen H, Zhu H, Zheng J, Mou D, Wan J, Zhang J, et al. Iontophoresis-driven penetration of nanovesicles through microneedle-induced skin microchannels for enhancing transdermal delivery of insulin. J Control Release. 2009;139(1) 63-72.

[41] Bariya SH, Gohel MC, Mehta TA, Sharma OP. Microneedles: an emerging transdermal drug delivery system. J Pharm Pharmacol. 2012;64(1) 11-29.

[42] Rao R, Nanda S. Sonophoresis: recent advancements and future trends. J Pharm Pharmacol. 2009;61(6) 689-705.

Chapter 7

Understanding the Effects of Roux-en-Y Gastric Bypass (RYGB) Surgery on *Type 2* Diabetes Mellitus

Raymond G. Lau, Michael Radin,
Collin E. Brathwaite and Louis Ragolia

Additional information is available at the end of the chapter

1. Introduction

Obesity is a grave public health concern in the United States today. From 2007 to 2008, the prevalence of obesity was over one-third of the U.S. adult population [1]. It contributes to significant morbidity and mortality including heart disease, stroke, cancer, arthritis and sleep apnea. *Type 2* diabetes mellitus (T2DM) also has been shown to increase with increasing obesity. Findings from the National Health and Nutrition Examination Survey (NHANES) (1999 – 2006) showed that nearly half of individuals with a body mass index greater than 40 kg/m^2 have diabetes [2]. Results from various studies have shown that weight reduction significantly reduces the risk of developing T2DM in obese individuals [3], as well as improving glycemic control in those already with T2DM [4,5].

Long term medical therapy for obesity is often unsuccessful for the majority of patients in clinical practice. Bariatric weight loss surgery has remained the most effective means of achieving and maintaining weight loss. More significantly, it has been shown to decrease mortality [6]. The Roux-en-Y gastric bypass (RYGB) is a type of bariatric surgery that involves the creation of a smaller stomach with a connection to the middle portion of the small intestine, bypassing the duodenum and a portion of the jejunum (see figure 1). Two limbs are created after the surgery. One limb, referred to as the alimentary or *Roux limb*, is where nutrient boluses pass from the stomach pouch. The other limb, which is the bypassed portion of the gastrointestinal tract, is known as the biliopancreatic limb. This limb transports secretions from the pancreas, liver, and gastric remnant. Most remarkably, many obese *diabetic* patients who undergo RYGB are relieved of their anti-diabetic medications in a matter of days. This improvement in glycemic control occurs before any significant weight loss [7].

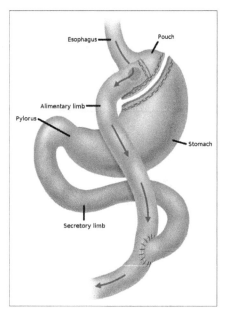

Dirksen C, Jorgensen NB, Bojsen-Moller KN et al. Mechanisms of improved glycemic control after Roux-en-Y Gastric Bypass. *Diabetologia. 2012*;55:1890-1901.

Figure 1. Roux-en-Y Gastric Bypass (RYGB)

This dramatic effect of gastric bypass on T2DM is not well understood. Improvement or remission of T2DM was thought to be due to weight loss in obese subjects [3, 5]. This was further supported by studies with gastric banding, a form of enforced caloric restriction [8]. However, clinicians began to observe that glucose levels were significantly lower in RYGB subjects as compared to weight matched controls [7]. Although malabsorption also likely contributes to the improved dysglycemia, there are other hormonal changes that are likely contributing to this effect. The most significant hormone changes occur in the secretion patterns of gut hormones. These are hormones that are secreted by enteroendocrine cells from the stomach, pancreas, and small intestine. A unique but significant post-prandial elevation of gut hormones is observed after RYGB. This is a well accepted phenomenon seen with RYGB subjects, and is believed to contribute significantly to this improvement of hyperglycemia in diabetics.

To better understand how RYGB affects those with *T2DM*, we will review the changes that occur with RYGB in key glucoregulatory organ systems within the body. In the ensuing sections, we will discuss in detail, the changes of *peripheral insulin sensitivity* and *insulin secretion* brought on by gastric bypass, and their effects on hyperglycemia. Identifying these changes will permit us to better understand how RYGB improves diabetes. We will also discuss the role that *caloric restriction* and *gut hormone elevation* may have in this process. Figure 2 demonstrates glucoregulatory variables that RYGB appears to modify. Cumulatively, this will permit the reader to develop an understanding of the relationship of how RYGB affects diabetes. We will begin our discussion describing the clinical potency of RYGB on T2DM.

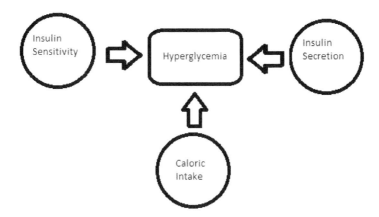

Figure 2. Glucoregulatory Variables

2. Problem statement: What is the effect of roux-en-Y gastric bypass on type 2 diabetes mellitus?

2.1. Roux-en-Y Gastric Bypass (RYGB) and its weight independent effect on T2DM

Since the early portion of the 21st century, there has been a growing interest in bariatric surgeries and their effect on ameliorating the diabetic state. Pories et al was arguably the first to describe remission of diabetes following gastric bypass. He reported gastric bypass not only caused weight loss, it also led to normalization of blood sugars in over 80% of his diabetic patients [9]. Initially, the normalization of blood sugars was thought to be directly caused by the weight loss. However, it has subsequently been noted that blood glucose control improves immediately following the surgery, prior to any significant weight loss. The concept that weight loss alone was not the reason for diabetes improvement after RYGB was a paradigm shift in the world of weight loss surgery, as well as the world of diabetes. This led to an explosion of research that attempts to understand how the surgery works.

There were few to no trials evaluating the efficacy of surgical treatment of obesity until the creation of the Swedish Obesity Study (SOS). The SOS trial is one of the largest prospective data collections to date that studies the clinical effects of various types of bariatric surgery. The SOS data demonstrates durable weight loss by as much 25% reduction at 10 years with various surgery types. The greatest weight loss is observed with RYGB [6] as compared to gastric

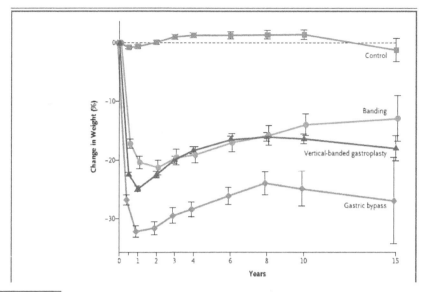

Sjostrom L, Narbro K, Sjostrom CD et al. Effects of bariatric surgery on mortality in Swedish obese subjects. *N Engl J Med.* 2007;357(8):741-52

Figure 3. Weight loss over 15 years between control groups (blue), gastric banding (orange), vertical banded gastro-plasty (purple), and gastric bypass (green).

banding, and a modified restrictive surgery known as vertical banded gastroplasty, (see figure 3). Since SOS, additional studies of obese subjects that have undergone RYGB have verified that weight loss from the surgery is durable and long lasting [10, 11].

While durability of the surgery continues to be validated in ongoing trials, its weight inde-pendent effect on diabetes was initially uncertain during the infancy of bariatric surgery. This uncertainty was at least partially due to the absence of appropriate "control groups" in various studies. For instance, the SOS data demonstrated reduced incidence of diabetes in surgically treated groups, but this was compared to non-standardized medically treated groups [12]. Medical weight loss therapy can be difficult to implement effectively, and therefore, compar-ison to surgical subjects is often imbalanced. This begs the question that if we can implement a medical treatment that *is as effective at achieving weight loss as gastric bypass, would we see similar improvements in diabetes?* Are there available studies that compare effective calorie restriction versus RYGB in terms of diabetes improvement? There are published studies using strict low calorie diets as a comparator group [13-15]. One such study by Plum et al demonstrated greater improvement in diabetes in RYGB subjects when compared to low calorie diets over three months [13]. Both groups had similar amounts of weight loss, suggestive that RYGB has weight independent effects on diabetes.

The surgical obesity procedure known as the gastric band may be perceived as a superior "control group" to dietary weight loss. The gastric band is an anatomically enforced form of caloric restriction and can be difficult to "cheat." Diabetes remission in subjects who had the gastric band has been shown to be directly related to weight loss, and was superior to conventional therapy programs [8]. However, prospective longitudinal studies comparing RYGB to gastric banding have demonstrated that RYGB promotes greater insulin sensitivity along with superior weight loss at one year [16]. Additional other types of studies have validated the potency of RYGB on diabetes through the use of other controls. One such study by Adams et al [17] was a large retrospective study of several thousand, comparing RYGB subjects to weight matched controls. This study demonstrated a remarkable 92% reduction in diabetes. Despite the overall lack of prospectively randomized control trials, there has been compelling data to demonstrate RYGB effectively treats hyperglycemia and the diabetic state.

Only in 2012 were the first prospectively, randomized, non blinded controlled studies made available, comparing weight loss surgery to medical weight loss therapy. Schauer et al [18] compared the RYGB and gastric sleeve surgical procedures to medical therapy in the STAM-PEDE study (Surgical Treatment and Medications Potentially Eradicate Diabetes Efficiently). Mingrone et al [19] compared RYGB and biliopancreatic diversion (BPD) procedures to medical therapy. The two studies had similar findings of greater "normalization" of glucose levels in the surgical patients as compared to medical therapy. However, there was still greater weight loss in the surgical groups, contributing to the greater glycemic improvement. Schauer et al [18] further demonstrated that the post-operative weight loss appeared to have no correlation with glucose control. This further highlights that RYGB has weight-independent effects on glucose control.

Both of the above discussed studies use *diabetes remission* as their endpoint. Before discussing the antidiabetic mechanisms behind RYGB, a further discussion of the meaning of *diabetes remission* will be explored. A seemingly simple concept, we wish to elaborate on the meaning of "diabetes remission," as well as discuss the associated complexities.

3. Application area: Can roux-en-Y gastric bypass be used to treat type 2 diabetes mellitus?

3.1. Roux-en-Y gastric bypass and remission of type 2 diabetes mellitus

Many subjects who undergo RYGB surgery and have T2DM observe a rapid normalization of their glucose levels, leading them to believe they have been "cured" of their diabetes. While these authors feel the term "cure" is incorrect, we cannot deny, and in fact pleasantly enjoy, watching the marked improvement in hyperglycemia following surgery. We agree that instead, the term *diabetes remission* should be used for these patients. Buse et al had [20] recently defined *prolonged diabetes remission* as hyperglycemia that is below the diagnostic threshold for diabetes for at least five years, while on no active pharmacologic therapy for diabetes. The increasing number of *diabetes remissions* after RYGB surgery has caused practitioners to revisit the definition.

Mingrone and Schauer's studies included similar definitions of *diabetes remission* in their trials, although their studies were less than five years in duration. Using diabetes remission as an endpoint acknowledges the potency of RYGB. But many questions come to mind amongst practitioners who manage diabetes. How does the surgery mediate such a potent effect? Should a reduced hemoglobin A1c be adequate for remission? Are the diabetic microvascular complications also reversed and should practitioners stop following these patients if they do go into remission? If there is complete reversal, why not use the term "cure?" Most important, has the characteristic pancreatic beta cell dysfunction reversed itself? These are questions proposed by these authors, some of which will be addressed in later sections.

Despite these questions, it is very hard to ignore the potent clinical effect the surgery has on diabetes. For those physicians and health care practitioners who struggle with uncontrolled diabetic patients, it is a seemingly effective and attractive solution. The metabolic potency of RYGB has even been addressed by the International Diabetes Federation (IDF) in a statement published in 2011 [21]. They discussed that bariatric surgery should be considered an option in those with a body mass index greater than 35 kg/m² and have T2DM. While a compelling argument can be made for this, we caution practitioners that not all RYGB subjects experience diabetes remission.

There are a small, but significant number of patients that have T2DM and undergo RYGB, but remain hyperglycemic post-operatively. In a retrospective review by DiGiorgi et al [22], as much as 24% of T2DM who had undergone RYGB had recurrence of their diabetes over a three year period, while a longer five year study demonstrated 31% recurrence [23]. Diabetes recurrence has also been seen as early three months following surgery [24]. These various studies demonstrated a number of factors that may contribute to recurrence. Higher BMI's, age, prior use of antidiabetic medications, and male gender were identified as factors associated with diabetes recurrence [23, 24]. A similar study in Chinese subjects demonstrated that diabetes duration, BMI, and fasting C-peptide were predictors for diabetes remission at one year. Based on this study by Dixon et al [25], suggestions of C-peptide above 2.9 ng/mL was a positive predictor for diabetes remission, which also implies residual good beta cell function within the diabetic group. These investigators were the first to suggest predictors and possible cutoffs in assessing the glycemic responses to RYGB.

Determining how to use RYGB in diabetes management is still in the early stages of development. Traditionally, this surgery was perceived only as a weight loss procedure. However, this has been an evolving paradigm within recent years. BMI alone is no longer the sole criteria for surgery in mildly obese subjects. Since 1991, the National Institutes of Health used both BMI and the presence of obesity-related comorbidities as the criteria for surgical weight loss. Even recent international guidelines still do not stray from these recommendations [26]. In the past, most studies looking at the effects of RYGB on diabetes have primarily focused on significantly obese subjects (BMI >35 kg/m²), although this is now changing. We have already pointed out that post-operative weight loss does not always seem to correlate with glycemic control [18]. A recent study by Cohen et al [27] examined people who had a lower BMI (30-35 kg/m²) and underwent bariatric surgery. They also demonstrated similar diabetes remission rates of 90%. Seeing such high rates of diabetes remission in a lower BMI range reinforces the concept of weight-independent effects of surgery on diabetes. As most obese individuals fall within this BMI range, clinicians may even consider recommending surgery at an earlier BMI.

Increasing evidence shows that BMI alone is not an adequate measure to predict successful health outcomes after RYGB. This is true for obese diabetics as well. We have mentioned that assessing for adequate beta cell function [25] could be used as criteria for successful diabetes remission. Additional evidence has suggested that those who have most benefited from surgery have elevated insulin levels, or insulin resistance [28, 29]. The simultaneous improved cardiovascular effects observed from the surgery [28] may also highlight the intrinsic relationship between insulin resistance and cardiovascular disease, often referred to as the metabolic syndrome. *As clinicians and scientists, it is critical for us to evaluate the effects of RYGB surgery beyond simple weight loss.* This may begin to help us stratify who best may benefit from the surgery. In the remaining portion of this chapter we will characterize the basic driving forces for T2DM and how the surgery brings about an improved glucose effect. This specifically will include *insulin sensitivity* and *insulin secretion*.

4. Observations and research: How does roux-en-Y gastric bypass improve Type 2 diabetes mellitus?

4.1. Effects of gastric bypass surgery on insulin resistance

Insulin action has a key role in regulating glucose homeostasis, facilitating glucose uptake in various tissue types. Its inability to cause glucose uptake is believed to be a key step in the pathogenesis of T2DM. This phenomenon is defined as insulin resistance. What mediates insulin resistance continues to be an active area of research. Glucose transport is maintained primarily through insulin-regulated glucose transporters, such as GLUT4. Commonly proposed theories that may mediate insulin resistance include impaired insulin signaling defects, GLUT transporter dysfunction, as well as increased availability of circulating free fatty acids. Both environmental and molecular factors may contribute to the development of insulin resistance. Obesity, as an environmental source, is believed to be a very common contributor.

Insulin resistance has been significantly observed at the level of the liver, skeletal muscle, adipose tissue, and pancreas. But it is skeletal muscle and adipose tissue that account for over 80% of total body glucose uptake. Because the reversal of diabetes immediately following gastric bypass is so profound, an alteration of peripheral tissue insulin sensitivity was thought to be the mechanism for achieving normoglycemia. With RYGB having superior weight loss, it has been well accepted that improved insulin sensitivity in surgical patients is also superior. However, the timing of when peripheral insulin sensitivity improves has been an area of uncertainty. Answering when peripheral insulin sensitivity begins after RYGB will also help to elucidate if it is a weight independent event.

The most frequently used measure of insulin resistance is the Homeostasis Model Assessment Insulin-Resistance (HOMA-IR). The ease of obtaining measurable glucose parameters have made this a popular method for quantifying insulin sensitivity. Several sources cite RYGB improves HOMA-IR from four days to two weeks following surgery in diabetic and non-diabetic subjects [30-31]. This is often before marked weight loss has taken place. In a non-weight controlled study, HOMA-IR was also decreased at three days following surgery [32]. However, these same sources demonstrate that HOMA-IR in RYGB subjects has comparable improvement to that of diet controlled subjects at similar time intervals while on calorie restriction [30-31]. Interestingly, there was minimal weight loss between the two study groups. *These findings are suggestive that immediate changes in HOMA-IR following RYGB are possibly related to caloric restriction alone.*

Besides HOMA-IR, there are other standard techniques for measuring insulin sensitivity. The gold standard remains the hyperinsulinemic euglycemic clamp. While most accurate in assessment of glucose uptake of *in vivo* systems, it requires experienced and skilled personnel often not readily available. The small body of literature that uses clamp data in gastric bypass subjects supports that insulin sensitivity in the post-operative period correlates with weight loss [31, 33], and therefore, is not a weight independent event in both diabetics and non-diabetics. Only Kashyap et al [34] demonstrated a slight increase of insulin sensitivity using clamp studies at one week following surgery for subjects that underwent gastric bypass as compared to gastric banding. However, as with all control groups, it is unclear if the oral intake of gastric band subjects was equivalent to the RYGB study group. Further molecular studies in rodent models that have undergone RYGB support the notion that insulin sensitivity is weight dependent. GLUT4 mRNA expression in skeletal muscle and adipose tissue of rodents that have undergone RYGB, does not increase until 28 days after surgery [35]. Therefore, the presence of adiposity reinforces the presence of insulin resistance. Because insulin clamp studies are the gold standard in assessment of peripheral insulin sensitivity, the *rapid glycemic improvement seen immediately following surgery appears not due to increased peripheral glucose uptake.*

Why there is this discordant finding between HOMA-IR measures and insulin clamp studies is unclear. Although HOMA-IR is an index of insulin sensitivity, it may also be used as a surrogate for hepatic insulin sensitivity. Therefore, one may observe there are more rapid improvements of hepatic insulin sensitivity than that seen with peripheral insulin sensitivity. However, there are only very few studies that intimately compare the two indices. HOMA-IR and peripheral insulin sensitivity were assessed through clamp studies, with individuals undergoing RYGB one month following surgery by Lima et al [36]. They demonstrated that there was no improvement of peripheral insulin resistance despite weight loss, although HOMA-IR did improve. Dunn et al used more dynamic and definitive methods for assessing hepatic insulin resistance using hyperinsulinemic euglycemic clamp studies with isotropic tracers, while also collecting data to asses for peripheral insulin resistance. They also demonstrated that there was also improvement in hepatic insulin sensitivity as compared to no improvement of peripheral insulin sensitivity at one month [37]. The reason for this requires further research.

Although RYGB and insulin secretion will be discussed in a later section, there are few studies that have measured hepatic glucose output in subjects that have undergone RYGB. Dunn et al [37] demonstrated decreased hepatic glucose production using clamp studies as described earlier. However, there was no appropriate dietary control group in this study. Contrary to these findings, Camastra et al [33] showed no improvement of endogenous glucose production one week following surgery against BMI matched controls. Because of these discrepant findings, the precise characterization of how RYGB affects hepatic glucose output also requires additional studies.

The clinical observation amongst practitioners in bariatric surgery is that in the immediate post-operative period after gastric bypass there is a rapid decrease of fasting glucose levels. However, dietary caloric restriction alone has been shown to decrease hepatic glucose output without affecting whole body glucose disposal [38-39]. People who undergo RYGB often have a post-operative decrease in appetite, anatomically imposed caloric restriction, and healing gastrointestinal anastomoses that require smaller nutrient boluses to allow for healing. In caloric restriction, the improvement of the endogenous glucose production (EGP) appears to be due to reduced glycogenolysis [40]. This finding is consistent with a study by Isbell et al [30] demonstrating comparable liver improvements (HOMA-IR) between RYGB subjects and calorie restricted subjects. Therefore, the rapid *alterations in hepatic metabolism seen immediately following gastric bypass may be from calorie reduction alone and not alterations brought on by the surgery itself.*

Further molecular studies have supported the notion that RYGB does not induce a weight independent effect on peripheral insulin sensitivity. Time-dependent GLUT4 expression in skeletal and adipose cells in rodents after RYGB and weight loss was discussed earlier [35]. Intramuscular lipid content has also been noted to decrease one year following surgery by as much as 44%, which also contributes to enhanced insulin action [41]. These observations alone suggest why peripheral insulin sensitivity is delayed and appears to be affected only by the presence of adiposity. Alteration in gut hormone levels have been strongly implicated as a cause for the metabolic improvement seen in RYGB subjects, but has not clearly been associated with the changes in altered insulin sensitivity. Glucagon-like peptide-1 (GLP-1) has been the most well studied of these gut hormones. The effect of GLP-1 on peripheral tissue has demonstrated some effect on glucose uptake in adipocytes and skeletal muscle cells [42-43]. However, the authors feel the effect of GLP-1 has more clinically significant effects on pancreatic function. The role of GLP-1 is discussed further in the section *"Identifying anti-diabetic factors of gastric bypass."*

It is of interest that RYGB and other weight loss surgeries have differential effects on insulin sensitivity and insulin secretion. The biliopancreatic diversion (BPD), a more malabsorptive surgery with a more extensive bypass, is often reserved for the super-obese population. However, this surgery been suggested to improve glycemia through normalization of insulin sensitivity [44]. This contrasts to RYGB, which we have discussed here, in that it does not appear to rely on insulin sensitivity for rapid improvement of hyperglycemia. We have demonstrated here that peripheral insulin sensitivity improves as a function of weight loss, independent of RYGB, whereas hepatic insulin sensitivity improves as a function of caloric restriction. Neural based mechanisms have also been implied as contributors to the glycemic improvement, although much is still not understood. This will be further discussed later in *"Other contributing factors to the anti-diabetic effect of RYGB."* We now will discuss how RYGB may affect pancreatic beta cell function, an essential hormonal regulator of glucose control.

4.2. Effects of gastric bypass surgery on pancreatic function

T2DM is characterized by both peripheral insulin resistance, as well as pancreatic beta cell dysfunction. For this reason, understanding how RYGB affects the pancreas may allow us to better understand why diabetes improves after the surgery. The majority of available studies involve dynamic biochemical measurements involving nutrient challenges. The impetus for study of these nutrient challenges, such as mixed meal testing, is based on the link between RYGB and postprandial gut hormone hypersecretion [45]. Exaggerated gut hormone secretion appears to occur because of the altered transit of nutrient boluses caused by the gastric bypass, and is a well accepted phenomenon. Several gut hormones have been suggested to also alter insulin secretion, and are termed "incretins." The *incretin* effect relates to the ability of an oral glucose load to result in an enhanced insulin response as compared to a similar intraveous glucose load. The distal gut hormone GLP-1 has been shown to be primarily responsible for mediating this effect, although other possible contributing anti-diabetic factors have yet to be characterized. There have been surprisingly few studies that have addressed the impact of RYGB on the release of insulin secretion and its relation to other gut hormones. We will first characterize the pancreatic secretory alterations brought on by the surgery, and then further explain associated hormonal and pancreatic cellular changes.

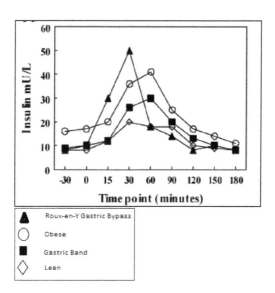

Le Roux CW, Aylwin SJ, Batterham RL et al. Gut Hormone Profiles following bariatric surgery favor an anorectic state, facilitate weight loss, and improve metabolic parameters. *Ann Surg.* 2006;243(1):108-14.

Figure 4. Roux-en-Y Gastric Bypass Insulin levels in Response to a Test Meal Le Roux C et al

Review of the descriptive studies of insulin secretion following RYGB suggest that fasting insulin levels appear to decrease within one week following RYGB in both diabetics and non-diabetics [32-34], which may be more of a function of improved hepatic insulin sensitivity. The majority of studies also demonstrate *a postprandial rise of insulin concentration that has a higher and earlier peak than seen pre-operatively* [32-34, 46-48]. While this suggests a possible restoration of the first phase of insulin secretion, this remains unclear. It also does not explain the exaggerated postprandial peak of insulin. The insulin peak also does not appear to be as marked as the postprandial GLP-1 elevations. The insulin peak is typically followed by a rapid decrease of insulin and glucose levels following the peak. This rapid decrease in levels is also not well explained. However, the insulin area under the curve (AUC), based on these prior studies, is either unchanged or decreased as compared to pre-operative measurements. Figure 4 demonstrates an example of post-prandial insulin levels in subjects that underwent gastric band and RYGB, as compared to control obese and lean subjects. The control obese subjects were matched to the pre-operative BMI of the surgical patients, and the subjects that underwent either operation had an equivalent post-operative BMI. Here, RYGB subjects exhibit the largest post-prandial insulin peak as compared to the gastric band and the remaining non-surgical subjects. Obese subjects likely have elevated insulin levels due to insulin resistance.

Decreased insulin levels following RYGB was generally believed to be the case with the perceived notion that insulin sensitivity was improved. However, as mounting evidence shows that peripheral insulin sensitivity is not immediately improved, these alterations in insulin secretion may hold more significance. Potential changes in alpha cell secretion of glucagon was then investigated to see if that had a possible role in these glycemic changes, namely if levels were decreased. However, they also had unexpected post-prandial elevations [48]. Why hyperglucagonemia would be present during the glycemic improvement seen after RYGB is unclear, and needs further studies to validate these findings.

Based on the postprandial insulin concentration profile demonstrated in figure 4, the glycemic effects do not clearly show why there would be an improvement of hyperglycemia. Available studies do not demonstrate consistently how postprandial glucose levels behave in response to these insulin secretory changes. Some have demonstrated significantly elevated postprandial glucose levels with a subsequent decrease [32], while others mostly show the postprandial decrease [8]. Inconsistency may have to do with varying nutritional content of test meals and timing after the surgery. Using other methods in assessment of glycemic changes with RYGB, continuous glucose monitoring (CGM) has revealed unusual patterns. In a group of RYGB subjects, CGM revealed increased glycemic variability using a calculation parameter known as "mean amplitude of glycemic excursions" (MAGE) [49]. The *increased glucose variability* may reflect an *altered postprandial insulin profile* that has been observed following RYGB, although this variability has only been identified in those afflicted with the condition known as *post-gastric bypass hypoglycemia* (*see Anti-diabetic effect gone too far? Postgastric bypass hypoglycemia* for further discussion). Studies into those RYGB patients without symptoms or documented hypoglycemia are ongoing. It is possible glycemic variability is a precursor to the metabolic complication *post-gastric bypass hypoglycemia*. Our laboratory is involved in trials studying this effect.

There are a greater number of studies examining the changes of insulin resistance in those that undergo RYGB and caloric restriction. There are far fewer studies comparing these two groups and assessing for differences in beta cell function. One study by Hofso D et al [50] compared RYGB to "intensive lifestyle intervention" as the nearest appropriate control. However, as expected, RYGB achieved superior weight loss, with significantly improved beta cell function. There are no available or appropriate weight matched trials to compare diet to RYGB on beta cell function.

The anatomic and histologic changes brought on by RYGB on the pancreas are also not well studied, due to the inability to easily access pancreatic tissue. The body of literature of known histologic or molecular changes within the pancreas that have been observed are restricted to rodent models, or those afflicted with post-gastric bypass hypoglycemia. One may expect hyperinsulinemia, especially in the setting of a marked peak in the postprandial insulin level. However, if the AUC of postprandial insulin levels are unchanged from prior to surgery, it is difficult to assess what cellular changes would occur if the same quantity of insulin was made by the beta cell. In rodents that have undergone RYGB, there has been a demonstrated increase in pancreatic beta cell area [51], less beta cell apoptosis [52], and increased beta cell proliferation [53]. This suggests that RYGB surgery enhances insulin secretion and insulin activity. However, as with all studies, appropriate controls are needed.

Much may also be learned of how RYGB affects the pancreas by the associated complication known as post-gastric bypass hypoglycemia (*reviewed further in"Antidiabetic effect gone too far? Post gastric bypass hypoglycemia*). Meier et al [54] demonstrated in human subjects who are afflicted with hyperinsulinemic post-gastric bypass hypoglycemia, the pancreatic beta cell area was not increased as compared to obese or even lean control subjects. They did demonstrate increased beta cell nuclear diameter in those afflicted with post-gastric bypass hypoglycemia compared to BMI-matched controls, suggestive of altered insulin production and secretion. One may therefore hypothesize that the decreased weight in response to the elevated insulin levels in RYGB subjects may be the responsible factor that improves glycemic control.

Despite these studies, further characterization is needed to understand how the pancreas responds to RYGB in T2DM independent of weight loss. Beta cell dysfunction is considered a hallmark of T2DM, often with hyperinsulinemia and gradual insulinopenia. This prompts the question of whether RYGB induces a reversal of these states. The altered post-prandial insulin profile seen after RYGB suggests beta cell function has only been altered, and not necessarily restored to appropriate physiologic function.

4.3. Identifying anti-diabetic factors of gastric bypass

Alterations of insulin secretion itself is a contributing factor that ameliorates the diabetic state in RYGB. Other contributing anti-diabetic factors brought on by RYGB are still being identified. Several investigators have proposed various intestinal mediators that may induce euglycemia, none of which have fully explained the clinical potency of RYGB.

Earlier studies suggested that exclusion of the proximal gut was responsible for the improvement of hyperglycemia, implying a potential "diabetogenic factor." Rubino et al [55] was the first to support this concept, by performing a duodenal-jejunal exclusion in diabetic rodents known as Goto-Kakizaki rodents. This was a surgery that led to preservation of gastric volume, with a pure exclusion of proximal intestinal absorptive surfaces. The initial excitement of his findings surrounded the premise that there was greater glycemic control as compared to calorie restricted rodents, simply by removing a portion of the intestine without creating caloric restriction. Born from this procedure was the concept of the "*foregut theory*." From this, it was perceived that there was a "diabetogenic factor" in this region of the intestine. However, this concept was later challenged by the "*hindgut theory*."

The "*hindgut theory*," perhaps more popular, operated on the premise that there were factors in the distal intestine that became elevated and had potent anti-diabetogenic effects. It is the author's opinion that this is the more likely theory. Further support for this are studies performed with feeding tubes placed in the gastric remnant of the intestine following RYGB. Hansen et al [56] demonstrated that using gastric feeding tubes led to increased gut hormones, as well as via oral (jejunal) routes. The similar alterations in insulin sensitivity between the two nutrient routes suggest the exclusion of nutrients from the foregut is not significant. Instead, distal gut factors such as GLP-1 may more likely be the cause.

GLP-1 physiology will not be covered here in depth. Its anti-diabetic effect in gastric bypass has been demonstrated in rodent models that underwent RYGB [57]. Research into GLP-1 led to drug development of GLP-1 receptor agonists. These agents are now in clinical use for the treatment of hyperglycemia. Its usage operates on the premise of augmenting beta cell function. Use of GLP-1 agonists or GLP-1 continuous infusions increased basal insulin secretion, often leading to an improved second phase of insulin secretion [58, 59]. Because fasting GLP-1 levels do not increase following surgery, many questions remain regarding its postprandial effects. Perhaps the most important evidence that there are other factors besides GLP-1 in RYGB that contribute to the anti-diabetic effect, is that the pharmacologic use of GLP-1 agonists have not led to the equivalent potency of RYGB surgery alone. This suggests there continues to be factors of the surgery that have still yet to be identified.

4.4. Other contributing factors to the anti-diabetic effect of RYGB

4.4.1. Roux-en-Y gastric bypass, satiety, and the central nervous system

The importance in assessment of decreased caloric intake with diabetes remission has already been discussed, in particular those that undergo gastric banding [8]. Similarly, the RYGB involves creation of a small stomach size, causing similar restriction. It is remarkable that subjects that undergo RYGB actually appear to have a markedly decreased appetite as compared to their gastric band counterparts. Because postprandial elevation of gut hormones is a distinguishing factor of RYGB from gastric banding, investigation of their orexogenic and anorexogenic tendencies have recently begun to be characterized. Earlier prospective studies generally demonstrated RYGB induced altered satiety [45, 60-62], although the field appears to be lacking trials that are appropriately controlled.

The evidence continues to mount for this gut brain communication effect, with several biochemical mechanisms that affect neural signaling of hunger and satiety being discovered.

Therefore, RYGB has effects on satiety that are *independent* of the physical limitations imposed by the formation of the gastric pouch. The effect gut hormones have on the neural circuitry are most studied specifically within the hypothalamus [63], with the balance of orexogenic and anorexogenic hormones. Prime hormonal candidates for these changes include insulin, leptin, GLP-1, peptide YY (PYY), and ghrelin [61-62, 64-65]. While findings with ghrelin have been mixed, there is growing evidence that the other aforementioned hormones may play a significant role. PYY [66-67] and GLP-1 [68-69] are currently being studied in great detail. Origins of these mediators come from multiple different organ systems, which subsequently affect neurons within the arcuate nucleus and other hypothalamic regions. These lead to alterations in food intake and body fat mass. Research into these anti-obesity mechanisms for pharmacologic uses are still being investigated.

4.4.2. Roux-en-Y gastric bypass, type 2 diabetes mellitus, and the central nervous system

Autonomic nerve regulation has often been the target for pharmacologic weight loss therapy. Therefore, there has been renewed interest in the role of the vagus nerve within bariatric surgical procedures to determine its role in weight loss. Preservation of the vagus nerve is a common practice by many bariatric surgeons. An intact vagus nerve with RYGB appears to have a significant and improved effect on food intake and weight loss [70]. However, the beneficial effect appears to carry over to improved glucose metabolism that also appears to be weight independent.

Obese and diabetic rodent models studies have demonstrated that hepatic vagotomy will worsen glucose metabolism [71-72]. This further highlights the necessary role of the vagus for helping attain euglycemia via hepatic-mediated mechanisms. This is not without some conflicting studies such as by Shin et al [73], although their focus was on food intake, body weight, and energy expenditure. Vagal signaling to the liver is mediated predominantly by parasympathetic fibers. These parasympathetic fibers are derived from the medio-basal hypothalamus. The source of this neuroendocrine regulation may suggest that hepatic glucose metabolism is uniquely regulated by a hypothalamic source.

Pocai A et al [74] demonstrated that activation of potassium-ATP channels within the hypothalamus appears to lower blood glucose through hepatic gluconeogenesis. This was a significant advance in better understanding the mechanisms that may mediate hepatic gluconeogenesis. Similarly, insulin presence near the hypothalamus has also been demonstrated to suppress lipolysis [75], which directly affects insulin resistance and T2DM. Additional characterization of the hypothalamic and vagal mediated effects may also help us to better understand the role of the nervous system in glucose and lipid regulation. Besides insulin, other hormonal candidates that were discussed earlier (e.g. PYY) may not only have anorexogenic effects that modify caloric intake, but they may also directly mediate glucose regulation via central nervous system mechanisms. Further identification of where gut hormone receptors exist are needed to better understand this potentially significant glucose-governing mechanism.

4.5. Anti-diabetic effect gone too far? Postgastric bypass hypoglycemia

Perhaps best described by the title of the article by Patti ME et al "*Hypoglycemia following gastric bypass surgery-diabetes remission in the extreme?*"[76] the condition of post-gastric bypass hypoglycemia has been an increasingly observed phenomenon. Contrasting mechanisms of how this occurs have been proposed, with the initial reports suggesting islet cell hyperplasia [77]. However, follow up studies suggested there was no change in beta cell mass, although there was an increase in beta cell nuclear diameter [54]. The increase in beta cell diameter may be more of a function of increased nuclear transcriptional activity of insulin production. This would coincide with those afflicted with this condition may have hypersecretion of insulin.

Hypersecretion of insulin at disproportionate levels to the decreased BMI following surgery may potentially lead to clinically significant hypoglycemia. This has been demonstrated in weight matched individuals by Goldfine AB et al [78]. If we recall the changes in peak of insulin secretion discussed earlier brought on by RYGB [32-34, 46-48], a comparison to BMI-matched subjects afflicted with hypoglycemia demonstrated a greater post prandial peak of insulin secretion [78]. This may lead to increased glycemic variability, which has been demonstrated in subjects who are afflicted with post-gastric bypass hypoglycemia [40].

While this is suggestive that RYGB may induce hypoglycemia via pancreatic mediated mechanisms, the question of the contribution of peripheral insulin sensitivity to hypoglycemia was answered by Kim et al [79]. Using intravenous glucose infusions in BMI matched controls, Kim et al [80] showed that those who are afflicted with hypoglycemia demonstrated appropriate insulin secretion rates in response to intravenous glucose challenges. Therefore, it appears the hypoglycemia is only brought on by ingestion of nutrient boluses which elicits an abnormal insulin response. While the response may be effective in mediating improved glucose control, it is unclear why some subjects develop hypoglycemia and others do not. Possible causes may have to do with prior history of diabetes and residual insulin resistance.

Because of the increasing number of bariatric surgeries being performed, this is an area that is in urgent need of further study. Understanding how this condition develops will also likely shed light on how the surgery helps improve hyperglycemia. Currently, our laboratory is involved with ongoing clinical trials to better understand the mechanisms behind this clinically significant phenomena.

5. Further Research: Can other weight loss surgeries help type 2 diabetes mellitus?

5.1. Sleeve gastrectomy: The future?

The growing popularity of the bariatric weight loss surgery known as the sleeve gastrectomy is worthy of discussion. The procedure involves the removal of the antrum of the stomach, with a creation of a sleeve-like structure. The potency of the sleeve gastrectomy on diabetes has been demonstrated by Schauer et al [18]. While the improvement of hemoglobin A1c reduction was greater in those that underwent RYGB, the sleeve gastrectomy had a similar reduction of almost 3% at one year following surgery. There was also a comparable reduction in BMI between the two surgeries. The question remains if there is a weight-independent effect of diabetes improvement with this surgery?

Earlier prospective studies of the sleeve gastrectomy, as compared to the RYGB, demonstrated that weight loss and glucose homeostasis was also similarly improved between the two [80-81]. However, they also demonstrated increased postprandial elevation of GLP-1, PYY, and insulin levels, although generally slightly less than RYGB. Short term (6 weeks) and long term (1 year) follow up demonstrated comparable GLP-1 responses to mixed meal challenges [82-83]. The alterations of GLP-1 and PYY secretion is confusing and remains not well explained within the literature. RYGB has been associated with earlier transit of nutrients to the distal intestine, stimulating an elevation of the "hindgut hormones." These elevations may potentially explain the glycemic improvement. However, these observations do not explain why the postprandial hormone elevation with the sleeve gastrectomy occurs. The literature still lacks a satisfactory mechanism of the stimulating mechanism for these elevations.

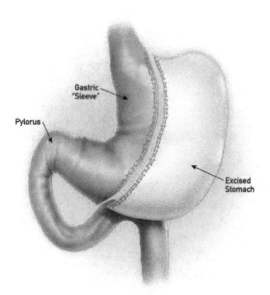

http://www.google.com/imgres?um=1&hl=en&client=tablet-android-asus-
nexus&sa=N&rlz=1Y3NDUG_enUS499&biw=1280&bih=699&tbm=isch&tbnid=MwIS5kgaHvl2BM:&imgrefurl=http://
www.ct-obesitysurgery.com/index.cfm/PageID/6424&docid=uP3rjSe-Kv1fMM&imgurl=http://ct-obesitysur-
gery.com//images_content/sleeve%252520gastrectomy.jpg&w=628&h=568&ei=DOyNUMC2NOPs0QHlzl-
CABQ&zoom=1&iact=hc&vpx=184&vpy=183&dur=122&hovh=213&hovw=236&tx=127&ty=142&sig=110329031745
694344091&page=1&tbnh=148&tbnw=164&start=0&ndsp=20&ved=1t:429,r:0,s:0,i:112

Figure 5. Sleeve Gastrectomy

It should be noted that most of these studies had small samples sizes and lacked appropriate controls. However, the clinical effects of the sleeve gastrectomy on diabetes remains difficult to ignore. The mechanism remains elusive, and many questions remain about the effects of the sleeve gastrectomy. Why do the post-prandial gut hormone elevations occur? What is the biologic mechanism? Is the surgery susceptible to the same post-surgery hypoglycemia seen with the RYGB? The increasing popularity of the procedure is for various reasons. The intact nature of the pylorus prevents the dumping phenomenon. The lack of an intestinal bypass prevents associated malabsorption and the plethora of micronutrient deficiencies. Lastly, the hypoglycemia phenomenon has not yet been reported with this procedure.

Despite these appealing features, we would advise practitioners to evaluate their patients carefully when considering a bariatric surgical method for weight loss. Little to no long-term studies are currently available on their clinical potency, and the lack of understanding how the surgery affects diabetes should give practitioners pause. However, the surgery is still very promising with apparently little metabolic complications. The authors are excited about the growing role of the sleeve gastrectomy in weight loss procedures.

6. Conclusion

RYGB unquestionably ameliorates the hyperglycemic state in many of those with T2DM. Many who undergo the surgery gain significant health benefits, and achieve remission of their diabetes. Investigators are attempting to understand the clinical impact of diabetes remission on RYGB patients, as well as the mechanism of how this is achieved. The improvement of peripheral insulin sensitivity appears to be weight dependent, while hepatic insulin sensitivity seems to be a function of caloric restriction. However, alterations in pancreatic function are reflected in the robust postprandial insulin secretion profile, and appear to be a direct result of RYGB. Understanding the condition of the pancreas' endogenous insulin producing ability and the whole body insulin resistance may allow us to predict who will achieve diabetic remission.

The increasing clinical phenomenon of post-gastric bypass hypoglycemia may be a result of an undesired overenhancement of the alterations brought on by surgery. This condition needs further study to better aide those afflicted with this potentially debilitating condition. As a possible alternative, the sleeve gastrectomy may potentially be an alternative weight loss surgery that appears to have lesser metabolic complications than are associated with RYGB. However, understanding of how it mediates its effect on diabetes is still not understood, and also is in great need of additional research.

Acknowledgements

We would like to thank Winthrop University Hospital for their support.

Author details

Raymond G. Lau[1], Michael Radin[2], Collin E. Brathwaite[1] and Louis Ragolia[3*]

*Address all correspondence to: lragolia@winthrop.org

1 Department of Bariatric Surgery, Winthrop University Hospital, Mineola, New York, USA

2 Department of Endocrinology and Metabolism, Winthrop University Hospital, Mineola, New York, USA

3 Department of Vascular Biology, Winthrop University Hospital, Mineola, New York, USA

References

[1] Flegal KM, Carroll MD, Ogden CL, Curtin LR. Prevalence and trends in obesity among US adults,1999-2008. *JAMA*. 2010;303(3):235-41.

[2] Nguyen NT, Nguyen XM, Lane J, Wang P. Relationship Between Obesity and Diabetes in a US Adult Population Findings from the National Health and Nutrition Examination Survey, 1996-2006. *Obes Surg*. 2011; 21(3): 351-5.

[3] Knowler W, Barrett-Connor E, Fowler SE et al. Reduction in the incidence of type 2 diabetes with lifestyle intervention or metformin. *N Engl J Med*. 2002; 346(6):393-403.

[4] Ross SA, Dzida GVJ, Khunti K, Kaiser M, and Ligthelm RJ. Impact of Weight Gain on Outcomes in type 2 diabetes. *Curr Med Res Opin*. 2011; 27(7):1431-8.

[5] Pi-Sunyer X, Blackburn G, Brancati FL et al. Reduction in Weight and Cardiovascular Disease Risk Factors in Individuals with type 2 diabetes: one year results of the look AHEAD trial. *Diabetes Care*. 2007;30(6):1374-83.

[6] Sjostrom L, Narbro K, Sjostrom CD et al. Effects of bariatric surgery on mortality in Swedish obese subjects. *N Engl J Med*. 2007;357(8):741-52

[7] Pories WJ. Diabetes: the evolution of a new paradigm. *Ann Surg*. 2004;239(1):12-13.

[8] Dixon JB, O'Brien PE, Playfair J et al. Adjustable gastric banding and Conventional Therapy for Type 2 Diabetes. *JAMA*. 2008;299(3):316-323.

[9] Pories WJ, Swanson MS, MacDonald KG et al. Who would have thought it? An operation proves to be the most effective therapy for adult-onset diabetes mellitus. *Ann Surg*. 1995;222(3):339-350.

[10] Edholm D, Svensson F, Naslund I et al. Long Term results 11 years after primary gastric bypass in 384 patients. *Surg for Obes and Relat Diseases*. 2012; [Epub ahead of print].

[11] Attiah MA, Halpern CH, Balmuri U et al. Durability of Roux-en-Y Gastric Bypass Surgery A Meta-Regression Study. *Annals of Surg*. 2012; 256(2):251-4.

[12] Sjostrom L, Lindroos AK, Peltonen M et al. Lifestyle, Diabetes, and Cardiovascular Risk Factors 10 Years after Bariatric Surgery. *N Engl J Med*. 2004;351(26): 2683-93.

[13] Plum L, Ahmed L, FebresG et al. Comparison of Glucostatic Pamaeters After Hypocaloric Diet or Bariatric Surgery and Equivalent Weight Loss. *Obesity*. 2011.; 19(11): 2149-57.

[14] Laferrere B. Effect of gastric bypass surgery on the incretins. *Diabetes Metab*. 2009;35(6 Pt 2): 513-517.

[15] Laferrere B, Teixeira J, McGinty J et al. Effect of Weight Loss by Gastric bypass Surgery Versus Hypocaloric Diet on Glucose and Incretin Levels in Patients with Type 2 Diabetes. *J Clin Endocrinol Metab*. 2008; 93:2479-2485.

[16] Korner J, Inabnet W, Febres G et al. Propsective Study Of Gut Hormone and Metabolic Changes after Adjsutable Gastric Banding and Roux-en-Y Gastric Bypass. *Int J Obes*. 2009;33(7):786-795.

[17] Adams TD, Gress RE, Smith SC et al. Long Term Mortality after Gastric Bypass Surgery. *N Engl J Med* . 2007;357:753-61

[18] Schauer PR, Kashyap SR, Wolski K et al. Bariatric surgery versus intensive medical therapy in obese patients with diabetes. *N Engl J Med*, 2012;366(17):1567-76.

[19] Mingrone G, Panunzi S, De Gaetano A et al. Bariatric surgery versus conventional medical therapy for type 2 diabetes. *N Engl J Med*. 2012;366(17):1577-85.

[20] Buse JB, Caprio S, Cefalu WT et al. How Do We Define Cure of Diabetes? *Diabetes Care*. 2009;32(11):2133-5.

[21] Dixon JB et al. Bariatric Surgery: an IDF statement for obese Type 2 diabetes. *Surg Obes Relat Dis*. 2011;7(4):433-47.

[22] DiGiorgi M et al. Re-emergence of diabetes after gastric bypass after gastric bypass in patients with mid to long term follow up. *Surg Obes Relat Dis*. 2010;6(3):249-53.

[23] Yamaguchi CM, Faintuch J, Hayashi Sy et al. Refractory and new-onset diabetes more than 5 years after gastric bypass for morbid obesity. *Surg Endo*. 2012;26(10): 2843-7

[24] Jurowich C et al. Improvement of Type 2 Diabetes Mellitus After Bariatric Surgery-Who Fails in the Early Postoperative Course? *Obes Surg*. 2012;22(10):1521-6.

[25] Dixon JB, Chuang LM, Chong K et al. Predicting the Glycemic Response to Gastric Bypass Surgery in Patients with Type 2 Diabetes. *Diabetes Care*.2012; [Epub ahead of print].

[26] Dixon AB, Zimmet P, Alberti KG et al. Bariatric Surgery: An IDF statement for obese Type 2 Diabetes. *Arq Bras Endocrinol Metab.* 2011;28 (6):628-642.

[27] Cohen RV, Pinheiro JC, Schiavon CA et al. Effects of Gastric Bypass Surgery in Patients with Type 2 Diabetes and Only Mild Obesity. *Diabetes Care.* 2012; 35:1420-1428.

[28] Sjostrom L, Peltonen M, Jacobsen P et al. Bariatric Surgery and Long Term Cardiovascular Events. *JAMA.* 2012; 307(1)56-65.

[29] Carlsson LM, Peltonen M, Ahlin S et al. Bariatric Surgery and Prevention of Type 2 Diabetes in Swedish Obese Subjects. *N Engl J Med.* 2012; 367:695-704.

[30] Isbell JM, Tamboli RA, Hansen RE et al. The Importance of Caloric Restriction in the Early Improvements in Insulin Sensitivity after Roux-en-Y Gastric Bypass Surgery. *Diabetes Care.* 2010;33(7):1438-1442.

[31] Campos GM, Rabl C, Peeva S et al. Improvement in peripheral glucose uptake after gastric bypass surgery is observed only after substantial weight loss has occurred and correlates with the magnitude of weight lost. *J Gastrointest Surg.* 2010;14(1):15-23.

[32] Falken Y, Hellstrom PM, Holst JJ et al. Changes in Glucose Homeostasis after Roux-en-Y Gastric Bypass Surgery for Obesity at Day Three, Two Months, and One Year After Surgery: Role of Gut Peptides. *J Clin Endocrinol Metab.* 2011; 96:2227-2235.

[33] Camastra S, Gastaldelli A, Mari A et al. Early and longer term effects of gastric bypass surgery on tissue-specific insulin sensitivity and beta cell function in morbidly obese patients with and without type 2 diabetes. *Diabetologia.* 2011;454:2093-2102.

[34] Kashyap SR, Daud S, Kelly KR et al. Acute effects of gastric bypass versus gastric restrictive surgery on B-cell function and insulinotropic hormones in severely obese patients with type 2 diabetes. *Int J Obes.* 2010;34(3):462-471.

[35] Bonhomme S, Guijarro A, Keslacy S et al. Gastric Bypass up-regulates insulin signalling pathway. *Nutrition.* 2011;27(1):73-80.

[36] Lima MM, Pareja JC, Alegre SM et al. Acute effect of roux-en-y gastric bypass on whole body insulin sensitivity: a study with the euglycemic hyperinsulinemic clamp. *J Clin Endocrinol Metab.* 2010;95(8):3871-5.

[37] Dunn JP, Abumrad NN, Breitman J et al. Hepatic and Peripheral Insulin sensitivity and Diabetes Remissionss at 1 Month afte ROux-en-Y Gastric Bypass Surgery in Patients Randomized to Omentectomy. *Diabetes Care.* 2012; 35(1):137-42.

[38] Jazet IM, Pijl H, Frolich M et al. Two days of a very low calorie diet reduces endogenous glucose production in obese type 2 diabetic patients despite the withdarwal of blood glucose lowering therapies including insulin. *Metabolism.* 2005;52:705-712.

[39] Kirk E, Reeds DN, Finck BN et al. Dietary fat and carbohydrates differentially alter insulin sensitivity during caloric restriction. *Gastroenterology.* 2009;136:1552-1560.

[40] Christiansen MP, Linfoot PA, Neese RA, and Hellerstein MK. . Effect of dietary energy restriciton on glucose production and substrate utilization in type 2 diabetes. *Diabetes* 2000;49(10):1691-1699

[41] Gray RE, Tanner CJ, Pories WJ et al. Effect of weight loss on muscle lipid content in morbidly obese subjects. *Am J Physiol Endocrinol*. 2003;284(4):E726-32.

[42] Villanueva-Penacarillo ML et al. Characteristics of GLP-1 effects on glucose metabolism in human skeletal muscle from obese patients. *Regul Pept.* 2011;168(1-3);39-44.

[43] Sancho V, Nuche B, Arnes L et al. The Action of GLP-1 and exendins upon glucose transport in normal human adipocytes, and on kinase activity as compared to morbidly obese patients. *Int J Mol Med*. 2007;19(6):961-6.

[44] Castagneto M, and Mingrone G. The Effect of Gastrointestinal Surgery on Insulin Resistance and Insulin Secretion. *Curr Atheroscler Rep*. 2012; 14(6):624-630.

[45] Borg CM, Le Roux CW, Ghaeti MA et al. Progressive rise in gut hormone levels after Roux-en-Y gastric bypass suggests gut adaptation and explains altered satiety. *Br J Surg*. 2006;93(2):210-5.

[46] Korner J, Bessler M, Inabnet W et al. Exaggerated GLP-1 and Blunted GIP Secretion are Associated with Roux-en-Y Gastric Bypass but not Adjustable Gastric Banding. *Surg Obes Relat Dis*. 2007;3(6):597-601.

[47] Laferrere B, Teixeira J, McGinty J et al . Effect of Weight Loss by Gastric Bypass Surgery Versus Hypocaloric Diet on Glucose and Incretin Levels in Patients with Type 2 Diabetes. *J Clin Endocrinol Metab*. 2008;93(7):2479-2485.

[48] Dirksen C, Jorgensen NB, Bojsen-Moller KN et al. Mechanisms of improved glycemic control after Roux-en-Y Gastric Bypass. *Diabetologia*. 2012;55:1890-1901.

[49] Hanaire H, Bertrand M, Guerci B et al. High Glycemic Variability Assessed by Continuous Glucose Monitoring After Surgical Treatment of Obesity by Gastric Bypass. *Diabetes Technology & Therapuetics*. 2011;13(6):625-30.

[50] Hofso D, Jenssen T, Bollerslev J et al. Beta Cell Function after Weight Loss: A clinical trial comparing gastric bypass surgery and intensive lifestyle intervention. *Eur J Endocrin*. 2011;164(2):231-8.

[51] Speck M, Cho YM, Asadi A et al. Duodenal Jejunal bypass protects GK rats from B-cell loss and aggravation of hyperglcyemia and increases enteroendocrine cells coexpressing GIP and GLP-1. *Am J Physiol Endocrinol Metab*. 2011;300(5):E923-32.

[52] Chai F, Wang Y, Zhou Y et al. Adiponectin Downregulates Hyperglycemia and Reduces Pancreatic Islet Apoptosis after Roux-en-Y Gastric Bypass Surgery. *Obes Surg*. 2011;21:768-773.

[53] Li Z, Zhang HY et al. Roux-en-Y gastric bypass promotes expression of PDX01 and regeneration of B-0cells in Goto-Kakizaki rats. *World J Gastro*. 2010;16(18):2244-2251

[54] Meier JJ, Butler AE, Galasso R et al. Hyperinsulinemic Hypoglycemia After Gastric Bypass Surgery Is Not Accompanied by Islet Hyperplasia or Increased B-cell Turnover. *Diabetes Care.* 2006;29:1554-1559.

[55] Rubino F, Marescaux J. Effect of Duodenal-Jejunal Exclusion in a Non-obese Animal Model of Type 2 Diabetes: A New Perspective for an Old Disease. *Annals of Surg.* 2004;239(1):1-11.

[56] Hansen EN, Tamboli RA, Isbell JM et al. Role of the foregut in the early improvement in glucose tolerance and insulin sensitivity following Roux-en-Y gastric bypass surgery. *Am J Physiol Gastrointest Liver Physiol.* 2011;300:G795-G802.

[57] Chambers P, Jessen L, Ryan KK et al. Weight Independent Changes in Blood Glucose Homeostasis After Gastric Bypass or Vertical Sleeve Gastrectomy in Rats. *Gastroenterology.* 2011;141(3):950-58.

[58] Nauck MA, Kleine N, Orskov C et al. Normalization of Fasting Hyperglycemia by Exogenous Glucagon-Like Peptide 1 (7-36) in Type 2 (non-insulin-dependent) Diabetic Patients. *Diabetologia.* 1993;36(8):741-4.

[59] Hojberg PV, Vilsboll T, Rabol R et al. Four Weeks of Normalization of Blood Glucose Improves the Insulin Response to Glucagon-Like Peptide-1 and Glucose-Dependent Insulinotropic Polypeptide in Patients with Type 2 Diabetes. *Diabetologia.* 2009;52(2): 199-207.

[60] Morinigio R, Moize V, Musri M et al. Glucagon-like peptide-1, peptide YY, hunger, and satiety after gastric bypass in morbidly obese subjects. *J Clin Endocrinol Metab.* 2006;91(5):1735-1740.

[61] Le Roux CW, Aylwin SJ, Batterham RL et al. Gut Hormone Profiles following bariatric surgery favor an anorectic state, facilitate weight loss, and improve metabolic parameters. *Ann Surg.* 2006;243(1):108-14.

[62] Le Roux CW, Welbourn R, Werling M et al. Gut Hormone as mediators of appetite and weight loss after Roux-en-Y gastric bypass. *Ann Surg.* 2007; 246(5):780-5.

[63] Korner J and Leibel RL. To eat or not to eat – how the gut talks to the brain. *N Engl J Med.* 2003;349(10):926-8.

[64] De Silva A, Bloom SR. Gut hormones and Appetite Control: A Focus on PYY and GLP-1 as Therapuetic Targets in Obesity. *Gut and Liver.* 2012;6(1):10-20.

[65] Korner J, Inabnet W, Conwell IM et al. Differential effects of gastric bypass and banding on circulating gut hormone and leptin levels. *Obesity.* 2006;14(9):1553-61.

[66] Chan JL, Mun EC, Stoyneva VA et al. Peptide YY levels are elevated after gastric bypass surgery. *Obesity.* 2006;14(2):194-8.

[67] Batterham RL, Cohen MA, Ellis SM et al. Inhibition of food intake in obese subjects by peptide YY 3-36. *N Engl J Med.* 2003;349(10)941-8.

[68] Gallwitz B. Anorexogenic effects of GLP-1 and its analogues. *Handb Exp Pharmcol.* 2012;209:185-207.

[69] Kanoski SE, Fortin SM, Arnold M et al. Peripheral and Central GLP-1 receptor populations mediate the anorectic effects of peripherally administered GLP-1 receptor agonists, liraglutide and exendin-4. *Endocrinology.* 2011;152(8):3103-12.

[70] Bueter M, Lowenstein C, Ashrafian H et al. Vagal Sparing surgical tehcnique but not stoma size affects body weight loss in rodent model of gastric bypass. *Obes Surg.* 2010;20(5):616-22.

[71] Milanski M, Arruda AP, Coope A et al. Inhibition of Hypothalamic Inflammation Reverses Diet-Induced Insulin Resistance in the Liver. *Diabetes.* 2012;61(6):1455-1462.

[72] Li X, Wu X, Camacho R et al. Intracerebroventricular Leptin Infusion Improves Glucose Homeostasis in Lean Type 2 Diabetic MKR Mice via Hepatic Vagal and Non-Vagal Mechanisms. *PLoS ONE.* 2011;6(2):1-7.

[73] Shin AC, Zheng H, Brethoud HR. Vagal innervation of the hepatic portal vein is not necessary for Roux-en-Y gastric bypass surgery-inducing hypophagia, weight loss, and hypermetabolism. *Ann Surg.* 2012:255(2):294-301.

[74] Pocai A, Lam TK, Gutierrez-Juarez R et al. Hypothalamic K(ATP) channels control hepatic glucose production. *Nature.* 2005; 434(7036):1026-31.

[75] Scherer T, O'Hare J, Diggs-Andrews K et al. Brain insulin controls adipose tissue lipolysis and lipogenesis. *Cell Metabolism.* 2011;13(2):183-94.

[76] Patti ME, Goldfine AB . Hypoglycemia following gastric bypass surgery—diabetes remission in the extreme? *Diabetologia.* 2010;53(11)2276-9.

[77] Service GJ, Thompson GB, Service FJ et al. Hyperinsulinemic hypoglycemia with nesidioblastosis after gastric bypass surgery. *N Engl J Med.* 2005;353:249-54.

[78] Goldfine AB, Mun EC, Devine E et al. Patients with Neuroglycopenia after Gastric Bypass Surgery Have Exaggerated Incretin and Insulin Secretory Responses to a Mixed Meal. *J Clin Endocrinol Metab.* 2007;92(12):4678-4685.

[79] Kim SH, Abbasi F, Lamendola C et al. Glucose-Stimulated Insulin Secretion in Gastric Bypass Patients with Hypoglycemic Syndrome: No Evidence for Inappropriate Pancreatic B-cell Function. *Obes Surg.* 2010;20:1110-1116.

[80] Peterli R, Wolnerhanssen B, Peters T et al. Improvement in Glucose Metabolism After Bariatric Surgery: Comparison of Laparascopic Roux-en-Y Gastric Bypass and Laparascopic Sleeve Gastrectomy: A Prospective Randomized Trial. *Annals of Surg.* 2009;250(2):234-41.

[81] Karamanakos SN, Vagenas K, Kalfarentzos F et al. Weight Loss, Appetite Supression, and Changes in Fasting and Postprandial Ghrelin and Peptide YY Levels afte Roux-

en-Y Gastric Bypass and Sleeve Gastrectomy: A prospective, Double Blind Study. *Annals of Surg.* 2008;247(3):401-7.

[82] Romero F, Nicolau J, Flores L et al. Comparable early changes in gastrointestinal hormones after sleeve gastrectomy and Roux-en-Y gastric bypass surgery for morbidly obese type 2 diabetic subjects. *Surg Endosc.* 2012;26(8):2231-9.

[83] Jimenez A, Casamitjana R, Flores L et al. Long-Term Effects of Sleeve Gastrectomy and Roux-en-Y Gastric Bypass Surgery on Type 2 Diabetes in Morbidly Obese Subjects. *Ann of Surg.* 2012;256(6):1023-9.

Chapter 8

Beneficial Effects of Alternative Exercise in Patients with Diabetes Type II

Additional information is available at the end of the chapter

1. Introduction

First of all, let's define the meaning of alternative exercise which means exercise activities aside from the ones that generally perform: running, walking, swimming, or biking [1]. This chapter provides reasons for encouraging alternative exercise to patients with diabetes type II. Moreover it provides knowledge of general modes of alternative exercise and their effects in diabetes and non-diabetes individuals. The exercise modes which are too difficult, aggressive, sports or normally performed such as swimming, cycling or running are not included. The clinical instruction such as indication or contraindication of the exercise is not described because it has already been mentioned elsewhere in this book. Moreover, other recommendation for these patients is well suggested in a previous study [2]. Finally, it described scientific knowledge of an alternative exercise i.e. Arm swing exercise (ASE) on improving glycaemic control and antioxidant activity in patients with diabetes type II. Further studies investigating the effects of ASE on other systems in patients with Diabetes Type II are needed.

2. Reasons for encouraging alternative exercise to patients with diabetes type II

Although moderate exercise (mostly are western style e.g. swimming, running or aerobic dance) at least 30 minutes of moderate-intensity exercise at least three days per week was recommended to prevent cardiovascular disease in diabetes patients [3], it is difficult to encourage them to these modes of exercise regularly. Alternative exercise is defined as various exercise modes performed alternatively e.g. Yoga, Martial Arts, TaeKwonDo and many others. Factors affecting the boring in exercise are intensity, equipment, complicated mode and duration. This alternative exercise should reduce boring and encourage people to do exercise regularly.

3. General modes of alternative exercise

This topic described many modes of alternative exercise which some of them are scientific proved in patients with diabetes type II but some are not proved.

3.1. Yoga

The word yoga means "union" in Sanskrit, the ancient Indian language [6].

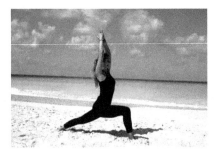

Figure 1. A posture of Warrior which is one of yoga positions [4]

Yoga is an old, traditional, Indian psychological, physical and spiritual exercise regimen that already has been known for its beneficial effects both the symptom and complication of patients with diabetes type 2 including;

• Decreasing reaction time [7]

• Improving lipid profile [7]

• Improving oxidative stress [8, 9],

• Can be incorporated along with the conventional medical therapy for improving cognitive brain functions in diabetes [8] and improve nerve function in mild to moderate Type 2 diabetes with sub-clinical neuropathy [10]

• Reducing Body mass index (BMI) and improving well-being [11]

• Reducing anxiety [8]

• Improving blood pressure, insulin, triglycerides and exercise self-efficacy indicated by small to large effect sizes. [12]

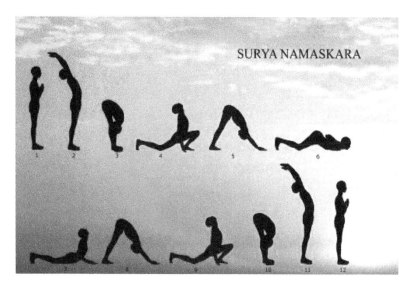

Figure 2. Postures of Surya Namaskara [5]

- Yoga-nidra with drug regimen had better control in their fluctuating blood glucose and symptoms associated with diabetes, compared to those were on oral hypoglycaemics alone. [13]

- Yoga asanas and pranayama improve glycaemic control and pulmonary functions [10].

Moreover, yoga practice was shown to improve pre-existing complication for those diabetic patients. Importantly, Yoga have a role even in prevention of diabetes. Yoga helps improving mind, body and spirit, leading to well-being and increased lovingly [15]. This may be due to mechanisms of reduction in stress and increase relaxations or noninvasive nature.

3.2. Bikram yoga

Bikram yoga is a system of yoga that Bikram Choudhury synthesized from traditional hatha yoga techniques [17] and popularized beginning in the early 1970s [18, 19]. Bikram Yoga sessions run for exactly 90 minutes and consist of a set series of 26 postures including 2 breathing exercises [20]. Bikram Yoga is ideally practiced in a room heated to 105°F (≈ 40.6°C) with a humidity of 40%,.

Bikram is a newer form of the practice that benefits blood circulation, improves cardiovascular conditioning and improves detoxification by increasing perspiration.

3.3. Koga

Koga combines the stretching and strengthening of Yoga with the cardiovascular workout of Kickboxing. Like yoga, Koga connects body with mind, and maintaining balance throughout.

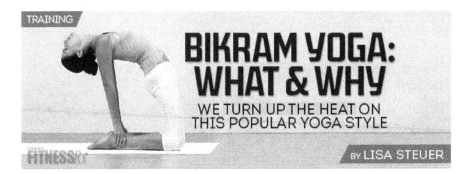

Figure 3. A posture of Bikram yoga [16]

Practicing Koga can help improve flexibility, increase muscle toning, relieve stress, increase lung capacity and decrease overall body fat.

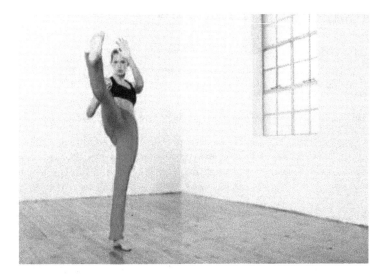

Figure 4. A posture of Koga [21]

3.4. Tai Chi

The Chinese characters for Tai Chi Chuan can be translated as the 'Supreme Ultimate Force' which is often associated with the Chinese concept of yin-yang, the notion that one can see a dynamic duality in all things. Tai Chi, can be thought of as a moving form of yoga and meditation combined. Many of these movements are originally derived from the martial arts although the way they are performed in Tai Chi is slowly, softly and gracefully with smooth and even transitions between them. Tai Chi is also situated in a wider philosophical context of Taoism. This is a reflective, mystical Chinese tradition first associated with the scholar and mystic Lao Tsu, an older contemporary of Confucius. He taught in the province of Honan in the 6th century B.C. and authored the seminal work of Taoism, the Tao Te Ching.

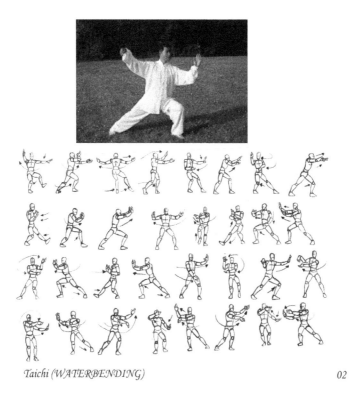

Taichi (WATERBENDING)   02

Figure 5. Postures and movements of Taichi [22]

Tai chi was shown to have many beneficial effects as the following;

- Improved indicators of health related quality of life (HR-QOL) including physical functioning, role physical, bodily pain and vitality in people with elevated blood glucose or diabetes who were not on diabetes medication [23]

- Improvements in fasting blood glucose and peripheral nerve conduction velocities [24].

- Improvements in physical and social functioning [25]

- Improvements in many parameters, such as BMI, lipid profile, C-reactive protein, and malondialdehyde [26]

- Preventing and improving psychological health and was associated with general health benefits for older people [27]

- Tai chi for those with type 2 diabetes could be an alternative exercise intervention to increase glucose control, diabetic self-care activities, and quality of life [28].

However, few studies did not support these beneficial effects of Tai chi [29]. Most of the studies are based on within group changes rather than attention control group comparisons [27].

3.5. Thai yoga (TY)

TY is a traditional form of exercise which appears to be a very light- to light-intensity exercise and have a low-impact alternative to jogging and walking for elderly individuals and requires no special equipment. TY may also have benefits in terms of stress management stemming from the meditation, relaxation and message aspects of the system. If individuals perform TY for longer duration especially standing position, they may gain benefits including reduction in cardiovascular mortality, reduction of symptoms, improvement in exercise tolerance and function capacity, and improvement in psychological well-being and quality of life [32].

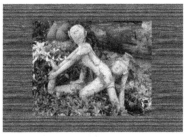 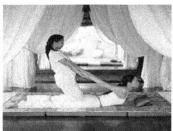

Figure 6. Postures of Thai yoga [30] [31]

3.6. Thai wand exercise

General health perceptions subscale of health related quality of life, functional capacity, body flexibility and obesity can be improved by Thai Wand Exercise training in older individuals [33]. This may partly reduce some cardiovascular disease risk factors. An advantage of this form of exercise is that this is a convenient, low impact on the joints and effective at home fitness program, with the only equipment need, a four feet long stick. But the major attraction is that it is also suited for the elderly who are not allegeable for the common training procedures.

3.7. Martial arts

Most people who are concerned with fitness often overlooked the martial arts. Besides learning to fight, it provides a true total body workout with improving core, upper and lower body strength. The core muscle generated the power in kicking and punching techniques. Impor-

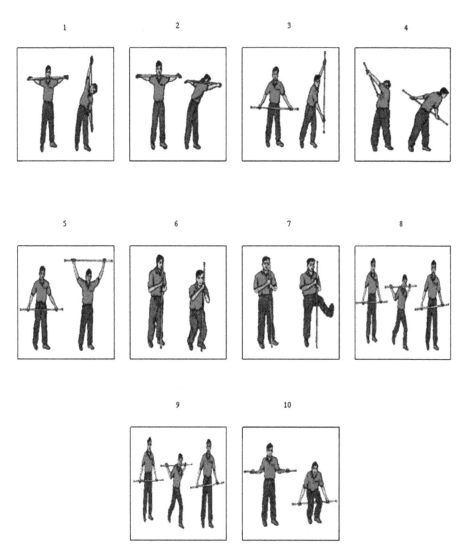

Figure 7. Postures and movements of Thai wand exercise

tantly, its training provides other benefits that are simply not found in an exercise class. First, it can help protecting someone from danger. It can also improve confidence and self-discipline which may change someone's life. Finally, it creates the friendships during training.

Example; Boxing-chaiya, Muay Thai, Chinese martial art, Judo, TaeKwonDo

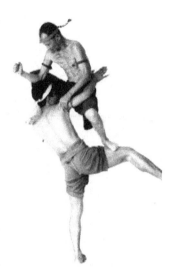

Figure 8. A posture of Boxing-chaiya [34]

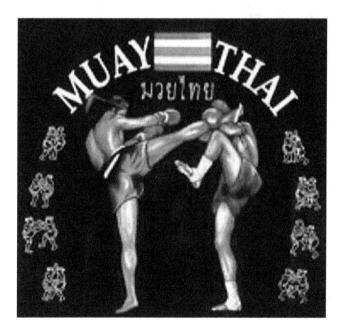

Figure 9. A posture of Muay Thai [35]

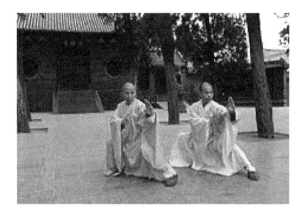

Figure 10. A posture of Chinese martial art [36]

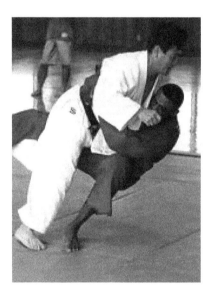

Figure 11. A posture of Judo [37]

3.8. Dancing

Dancing burns 2015 kilojoules an hour. It was shown to reduce risks for heart disease and diabetes in elementary school children [41]. Dancing 2 times per week for 12 weeks can reduce systolic BP and body fat in diabetes [42].

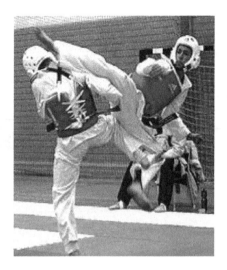

Figure 12. A posture of Taekwondo [38]

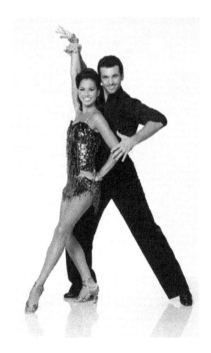

Figure 13. A posture of dancing [39]

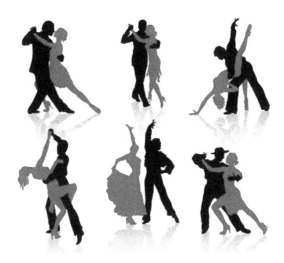

Figure 14. Postures of dancing [40]

3.9. Walking

Walking is recommended for preventing or treating diabetes patients [43]. However, walking with others can actually help patients stick with their health and fitness goals [44].

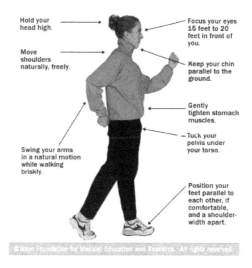

Figure 15. Detail of various postures and movements during walking

3.9.1. Brisk walking

The prescription of brisk walking represents an equally effective intervention to modulate glycaemic control and cardiovascular risk profile in type 2 diabetes patients when compared with more individualised medical fitness programmes. The Centers for Disease Control and Prevention (CDC) defined that brisk walking is at a pace of three miles per hour or more (but not race walking) or roughly 20 minutes per mile. This equates to about five kilometers per hour or 12 minutes per kilometer [45]. The exercise intensity of Brisk walking is moderate which heart rate is about 50-70% maximum heart rate or shouldn't be able to sing.

3.10. Go Ape

An exciting range of forest-based high-wire activities, comprise challenging courses that involve climbing, zip wires, balance beams and a whole range of fun-filled activities [47].

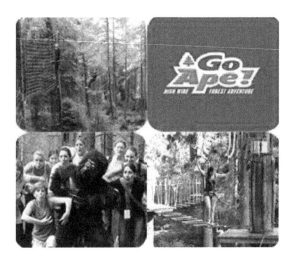

Figure 16. Different activities of Go Ape [46]

This activity lasts for 2 to 3 hours which some stamina to complete the course is needed. Upper body and legs will get benefit from this activity. Arm and leg flexibility will be maintained stretching and reaching for hand-holds along the course. Coordination will be definitely improved because of continually coordinating hands and feet as traverse the various obstacles.

3.11. Dinghy sailing

Dinghy sailing is the activity of sailing small boats by using five essential controls: [47]

• The sails

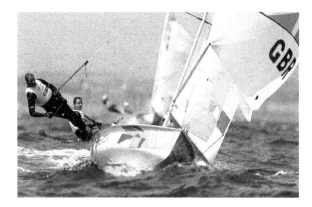

Figure 17. Movement of the crew during Dinghy sailing [48]

- The foils (i.e. the daggerboard or centreboard and rudder and sometimes lifting foils as found on the Moth).

- The trim (forward/rear angle of the boat in the water)

- Side to side balance of the dinghy by movement of the crew, particularly in windy weather ("move fast or swim").

- The choice of route (in terms of existing and anticipated wind shifts, possible obstacles, other water traffic, currents, tides etc.).

Dinghy sailing increases stamina because of the vigorous sailing especially shifting position to balance the boat. Rigging and de-rigging to hauling on the sheets increase upper body strength. Additionally, if there is a less stable boat situation abdominal and back muscles will be stimulated. Good flexibility is very necessary for dinghy sailing. Having a good range of movement and being able to stretch during balancing against the wind is vital. Successful small boat sailing requires because of frequently hauling on the sheets, tacking, shifting position and balancing all at the same time. This will certainly improve coordination.

3.12. Horse riding

Training of horse riding can increase insulin sensitivity in patients with diabetes type 2 [51, 52].

Generally, horse riding increases stamina according to maintaining an upright posture while continually controlling a moving horse at speed. It also strengthens core muscles in order to control horse's movements while maintaining an upright posture. However, there are few flexibility benefits from horse riding, but a good measure of all-round mobility to successfully riding is still needed. Coordination is important for marrying up small body movements with control of the reins — plus hand-to-eye coordination will be required during negotiating trails and obstacles [47].

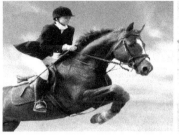
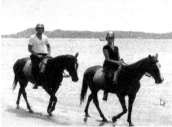

Figure 18. Upright postures during Horse riding [49] [50]

3.13. Fishing

During fishing, endurance is important for spending the best part of a day standing in a river, walking up and down a beach or fighting with a really big specimen for a few hours. Leg strength is increased from continually working a fly at full stretch. Casting a line is a skill that needs excellent arm and shoulder flexibility so upper body flexibility in particular will be improved by fishing. Casting the line and controlling the rod when reeling fish in requires good hand-to-eye coordination.

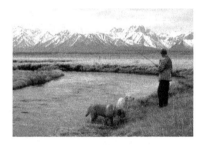

Figure 19. Standing posture during Fishing [53]

3.14. Lunge walking

The following is the movement of Lunge walking [54]:

- Stand upright, feet together, holding two light (5-8 pound) dumbbells at your sides (palms facing in).

- Take a controlled step forward with your left leg.

- Lower hips toward the floor and bend both knees (almost at 90 degree angles). The back knee should come close but never touch the ground. Your front knee should be directly over the ankle and the back knee should be pointing down toward the floor.

- Push off the weight with your right foot and bring it forward to starting position (#1). This completes one rep.

- Next step forward and repeat with the right leg.

- Do 2 sets of 15 reps.

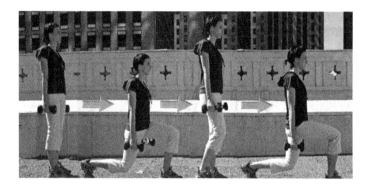

Figure 20. Series of movements of Lunge walking [54]

3.15. Make the most of the outdoors

Activities outdoors such as park benches, the kerb, and stairs for simple exercises are health benefit according to exposure to sun shine.

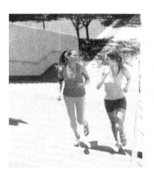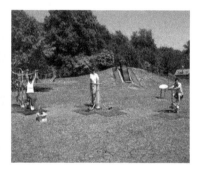

Figure 21. Activities outdoors such as park benches, and stairs [55] [56]

3.16. Surf

Feel the sun on your face and the thrill of catching waves along beautiful coastlines.

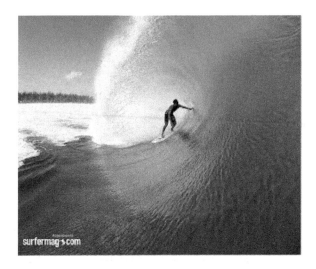

Figure 22. A posture under the wave during surfing [57]

3.17. Cardio tennis

Cardio Tennis is a new kind of group exercise that combines endurance with tennis skills. It includes thinking how to hit a backhand, followed by footwork exercises on a rope ladder and running drills. Then it's back to the volley line and hitting balls again. It was started in the US by the Tennis Industry Association as a way to get more people into tennis, but the programme has since rolled out to 1500 work-out sites in 25 countries.

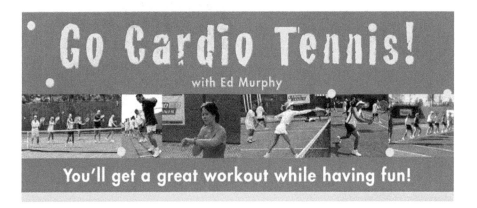

Figure 23. Activities of Cardio Tennis [58]

Each class includes 5-10 minutes warm-up segment including stretching and footwork drills and 50-55 minutes cardio segment including fun drills [58].

It provides:

• Much more fun than working out on a machine

• It's a fun group activity for advanced beginner and above players

• Elevate your heart rate into your aerobic training zone

• The focus is on getting a great workout while having fun!

3.18. Housework

Housework is so useful because it both increases energy expenditure, cardiovascular response and tidy a house. But if someone have balance problems, they must be careful going downstairs. It's very easy to fall, especially when carrying a vacuum cleaner. Whenever you see a set of stairs, use them. If there's time (and you're really enthusiastic), go back down and climb them again. If flexibility and balance aren't an issue, take two steps at a time.

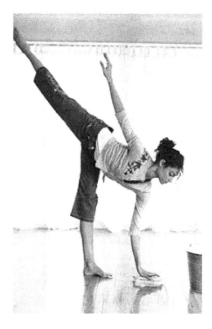

Figure 24. A posture of Housework [59]

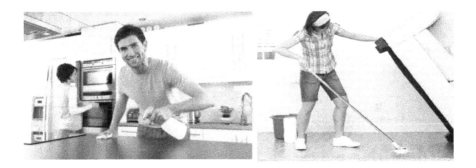

Figure 25. Activities of Housework [60] [61]

3.19. Alexander technique

Invented by an Australian in the 1890s, this technique helps to restore the body's capacity for ease by releasing tension, particularly in the head and neck. It aims to allow the body to reach its full potential.

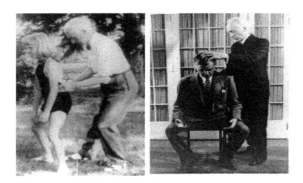

Figure 26. Alexander Technique [62]

"The Alexander Technique is a way of learning to move mindfully through life. The Alexander process shines a light on inefficient habits of movement and patterns of accumulated tension, which interferes with our innate ability to move easily and according to how we are designed. It's a simple yet powerful approach that offers the opportunity to take charge of one's own learning and healing process, because it's not a series of passive treatments but an active exploration that changes the way one thinks and responds in activity. It produces a skill set that can be applied in every situation. Lessons leave one feeling lighter, freer, and more grounded." [62]

The Alexander technique has been shown to be helpful for back pain and Parkinson's [63].

3.20. Feeldenkrais method

Developed in the 1940s, Moshé Feldenkrais (1904–1984) is a practical discipline to help develop awareness of body movement [65]. Feldenkrais aims to reduce pain or limitations in movement, to improve physical function, and to promote general wellbeing by increasing students' awareness of themselves and by expanding students' movement repertoire [66].

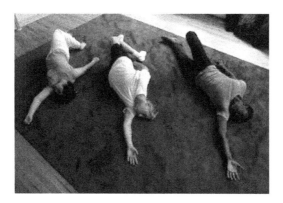

Figure 27. A posture of Feeldenkrais method [64]

3.21. Pilates

Invented in the early 20th century by Joseph Pilates, Pilates combines East and West, gymnastic and yogic principles, mind and body [70]. Pilates is a body conditioning routine that may help build flexibility, muscle strength, and endurance in the legs, abdominals, arms, hips, and back. It puts emphasis on spinal and pelvic alignment, breathing, and developing a strong core or center, and improving coordination and balance. Pilates' system allows for different exercises to be modified in range of difficulty from beginning to advance. Intensity can be increased over time as the body conditions and adapts to the exercises [71].

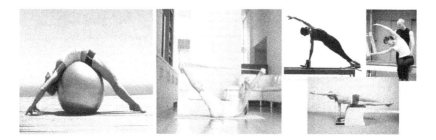

Figure 28. Postures of Pilates [67] [67] [68]

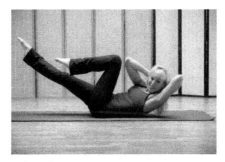

Figure 29. A posture of Pilates [69]

4. Beneficial effects of arm swing exercise on glycaemic control and oxidative stress in patients with diabetes type II [72]

4.1. Introduction

Although moderate exercise (mostly are western style e.g. swimming, running or aerobic dance) at least 30 minutes for five days per week was recommended to prevent cardiovascular disease in diabetes patients [2], it is difficult to encourage them to exercise regularly. Many Asian styles of exercise such as arm swing exercise seem to be more appropriate because of its simple, low impact to joint and easily accessible exercise.

Arm Swing Exercise (ASE) is a traditional Chinese exercise [73] which is convenient for diabetes patients to perform. It is believed to improve cardiovascular systems. However there were no scientific data concerning the beneficial effect and mechanism of this exercise on the glycaemic control. Therefore, this study aimed to investigate effects of the ASE training on blood glucose (glycated haemoglobin; HbA_{1c}), oxidant (determined by malondialdehyde; MDA) and antioxidant (determined by glutathione; GSH) in subjects with type 2 diabetes.

4.2. Experimental design and protocol

All subjects performed 2 study periods consecutively; i) maintaining daily life without regular exercise for 8 weeks (week 1-8) ii) performing 30-min ASE per day, 3 days per week for 8 weeks (week 9-16). Fasting blood glucose, HbA_{1c}, insulin, lipid profiles, C reactive protein (CRP), MDA and reduced GSH concentrations were analyzed using blood samples collected from the antecubetal vein. Anthropometry and body composition were also measured before and after of each study period. HbA_{1c} was used to determine glycaemic control because it is more stable throughout 2-3 months and related to the complications.

Insulin sensitivity was determined using Homeostatic Model Assessment – Insulin Resistance (HOMA-IR) [74]. Pharmacology, dietary and exercise treatment, were not modified during the study period. During the exercise period, patients performed the ASE program as prescribed. They were requested to record the 24-hour dietary composition and energy expenditure for 2 weekdays and 1 weekend day before the start and the last week of each period.

4.3. Arm Swing Exercise (ASE)

ASE is a traditional Chinese exercise which has been practiced for 50 years (Figure 1) and claimed for treatment of cancer and alimentary disorders by increasing blood flow [73]. The number of swing was 200 or 300 repetitions in the beginning and gradually increased to 1000-2000 repetitions or up to half an hour depending on the strength of the patients. The intensity of ASE is mild because it was around 23 percentage of maximal oxygen consumption and 45 percentage of maximal heart rate.

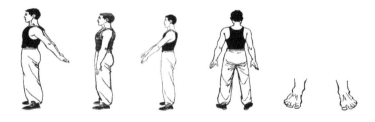

Figure 30. Postures and movements of body during the ASE

During ASE period participants learned to perform the ASE correctly on the first day of the experiment. For the next 8 weeks they performed the training at home via a video tape recording one session per day (30 minutes), 3 days/week. Each participant was telephoned every week to check their compliance to the program and to emphasize them to maintain their usual daily physical activity apart from the ASE program.

4.4. Statistical analysis

All dependent variables were analyzed using a two-way ANOVA with repeated measures (within subject factors were exercise and time) by Sigma Stat version 2 program. The Bonferroni method was used to adjust the multiple comparisons. A probability of $p < 0.05$ was taken to indicate significance. Results are presented as means SE.

4.5. Results

Nine male and 33 female patients with type 2 diabetes mellitus completed the study. Before the experiment, they had high cardiovascular risks such as hyperglycaemia, overweight or obesity (based on criteria of World Health Organization Western Pasific region), high fasting blood glucose, haemoglobin A1c (HbA_{1c}), high sensitive C reactive protein (hsCRP), MDA and low reduced glutathione (GSH) concentrations. There were no differences in body mass, body mass index, fat mass, fat free mass, waist circumference, hip circumference, waist to hip circumference ratio, and physiological characteristics between the two periods. Mean daily dietary intakes were similar in both periods (1,468.6 ± 58.6 kJ and 1,462.2 ± 56.0 kJ; control and exercise periods, respectively). Mean energy expenditure in the exercise period was significantly higher than that in the control period (1,593.4 ± 54.6 and 1,472.7 ± 47.6 kJ, respectively; p<0.05).

4.6. Clinical chemistry

HbA_{1c} concentration was 0.2% lower after ASE training for 8 weeks compared with the control period (p<0.05, Table 1). However, there was no significant difference in fasting blood glucose between periods. There were no effect of ASE training on insulin sensitivity, hsCRP concentration and lipid profiles between periods

4.7. Oxidative stress

ASE training significantly reduced plasma MDA concentration (p<0.05) and increased antioxidant blood GSH concentration (p<0.05). No correlation between oxidative stress and HbA_{1c} at any periods was found.

4.8. Discussion

The results showed that the ASE training improves glycaemic control and oxidative stress in patients with type 2 diabetes. Thus, this simple and accessible exercise may have a potential effect on the prevention of complications of diabetes mellitus.

Previous studies also found the decreased HbA_{1c} after the arm exercise training [75-77]. Jeng et al (2002) have reported that arm exercise training for 10-40 min could induce a significant decrease in the HbA_{1c} concentration in patients with type 2 DM. Data from the United Kingdom Prospective Diabetes Study Group (UKPDS) have suggested that a 1% rise in HbA_{1c} concentration represents a 37% increased risk for microvascular complications (95% CI 33 to 41, P < 0.0001) [78]. Based on this information, a 0.2% decrease in HbA_{1c} after the ASE training detected in this study may reduce 7.4% of risk for microvascular complications.

Possible mechanisms that could explain for the benefit effect of the ASE training on improving glycaemic control include the reduced HbA_{1c} and the effect of exercise per se on improving the oxidative stress. The reduced HbA_{1c} may decrease many adverse effects of hyperglycaemia such as hyperglycaemia-induced glucose autoxidation, non-enzymatic glycation of proteins, and reactive oxygen species generation, in leading to the progression of diabetic vascular complications. These processes were shown to increase oxidant stress and decrease antioxidant agent [79-81]. The imbalance of oxidative stress with greater oxidant stress contributed to the cellular destruction and therefore vascular complications [82]. The decreased MDA found in this study indicated a reduction in lipid peroxidation, a process of oxidative stress, which then reflects an attenuation of the cellular damage in the patients. The increased level of non-enzymatic antioxidant GSH after the ASE training observed in the present study also supports the preventive effect of exercise on vascular complication. As found in the present study, the improved glycaemic control positively indicate a preventive action of ASE training in the vascular complications in type 2 diabetic patients via the improved oxidative stress [82].

The second mechanism is due to the effect of exercise per se on improving the oxidative stress. This is supported by the absence of relationship between HbA_{1c} and MDA and GSH at any periods in this study. Importantly, this may remind that only improvement of HbA_{1c} from medication or diet control may not be enough to prevent the complication. Previous studies in both animal and human also supports that low-intensity exercise could itself improve oxidative stress [83-86]. Moien-Afshari et al have confirmed that the low-intensity exercise could enhance antioxidant agent giving rise to less endothelial dysfunction independently on the improvement of hyperglycaemia.

The present study showed that ASE has no adverse effects such as exercise-related injury or hypoglycaemia. This was shown by the similar level of CRP in both periods. Therefore ASE is appropriate and safe for the patient with diabetes. The other strength of the present study is a study design which each subject performed both control and exercise periods. This eliminates the effect of inter-individual variation.

4.9. Conclusion

In conclusion, the present study showed that the ASE training, a low-intensity exercise contribute to protective effects on vascular complication which is a major problem of type 2 diabetic patients. This may attribute to an improved oxidative stress according to either improved glycaemic control or exercise per se. The major attraction is that it is suited for not only diabetic patients but also other people who are not allegeable for the common training procedures such as elderly adults and patients with lower limb disorders.

5. Beneficial mechanisms of exercise on type 2 diabetic patients

There are many possible mechanisms explaining the beneficial effects of exercise training on type 2 diabetic patients (T2D).

These are described based on their roles.

6. Improve glucose control

6.1. Insulin-independent mechanism

1. Exercise leads to an insulin independent increase in glucose transport, mediated in part by AMP activated protein kinase. Changes in protein expression may be related to increased signal transduction through the mitogen-activated protein kinase (MAPK) signaling cascades, a pathway known to regulate transcriptional activity [87].

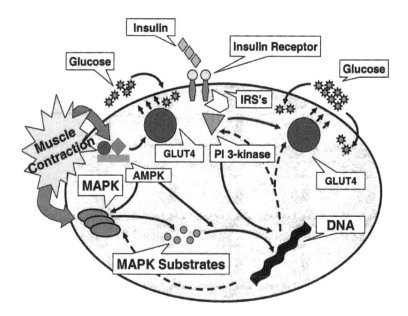

Figure 31. Exercise training-induced changes in insulin signaling via insulin-independent pathway in skeletal muscle [87].

2. Exercise increased skeletal muscle c-Jun N-terminal kinase (JNK) activity throughout the experiment, whereas insulin did not significantly increase JNK activity. The p38 activity was slightly stimulated by exercise and not by insulin [88]. However, the other previous study noted that exercise training improves basal glucose metabolism without a change in the stress kinases, JNK, the nuclear factor B (NF-B) pathway and Hsp72. Moreover, nuclear regulation of NF-B activity in diabetic muscle could be regulated independently of the cytosolic pathway [89].

3. The sodium-dependent glucose co-transporter system (hSGLT3), an insulin-independent glucose transporter, is activated by exercise and it may play a significant role in improving glycemic control [90].

4. Exercise training increases insulin-stimulated glucose disposal primarily by increasing GLUT4 protein expression without enhancing insulin-stimulated PI 3-kinase signaling, and that once the glucose enters the myocyte, increased glycogen synthase activity preferentially shunts it into glycogen synthesis [91].

6.2. Insulin dependent mechanism

The beneficial effect of exercise training on the control of glucose via insulin signaling has been reviewed by many previous studies [92-94]. In addition, many studies investigated the effects of exercise

1. More recent observations indicate that interactions exist at the distal signaling level of AS160 and atypical protein kinase C (aPKC) [95].

2. Acute exercise reverses TRB3 expression and insulin signaling restoration in muscle. Thus, these results provide new insights into the mechanism by which physical activity ameliorates whole body insulin sensitivity in type 2 diabetes [96]. TRB3 is an inducible gene whose expression is regulated by stress response and insulin and associated with insulin resistance and metabolic syndrome.

3. Exercise training increases skeletal muscle Nicotinamide phosphoriboxyltransferase (NAMPT) which is known as pre-B-cell colony-enhancing factor 1 (PBEF1) or visfatin, is an enzyme belonging to the family of glycosyltransferases, to be specific, the pentosyl-transferases. NAMPT was reported to be an activate insulin receptor and has insulin-mimetic effects, lowering blood glucose and improving insulin sensitivity [97].

4. Blood glucose concentration can be improved by exercise training-induced increases in muscle glycogen content. This could be regulated by multiple mechanisms, including enhanced insulin sensitivity, glycogen synthase expression, allosteric activation of glycogen synthase, and PP1 activity [98]. The increased muscle glycogen also plays important role in muscle strength [99]. This can improve glucose uptake and then glucose control.

5. Exercise overrules free fatty acid-mediated inhibition of pyruvate dehydrogenase (i.e., carbohydrate oxidation). This may improve carbohydrate oxidation although high fat was ingested [100]. The improved carbohydrate oxidation then enhances insulin sensitivity resulting in improved glucose control.

6. The metabolic outcomes were divided into six domains: glycogen, glucose facilitated transporter 4 (GLUT4) and insulin signaling, enzymes, markers of inflammation, lipids metabolism and so on. Beneficial adaptations to exercise were seen primarily in muscle fiber area and capillary density, glycogen, glycogen synthase and GLUT4 protein expressions [101]. This adaptation then play important role on improved glycaemic control.

7. Exercise training results in a persistent increase in insulin sensitivity in skeletal muscle from obese and insulin-resistant individuals [102]. Chronic exercise upregulated phosphorylation and expression of AMPK upstream kinase, LKB1. Particularly exercise reversed the changes in protein kinase C (PKC)ζ/λ phosphorylation, and PKCζ phosphorylation and expression. In addition, exercise also increased protein kinase B (PKB)/Akt1, Akt2 and GLUT4 expression, but AS160 protein expression was unchanged. Chronic exercise increased Akt (Thr (308)) and (Ser(473)) and AS160 phosphorylation. Finally, exercise increased peroxisome proliferator-activated receptor-γ coactivator 1 (PGC1) mRNA expression in the soleus of diabetic rats. These results indicate that both chronic and acute exercise influence the phosphorylation and expression of components of the AMPK and downstream to PIK3 (aPKC, Akt), and improve GLUT4 [103].

8. Exercise training reversed abnormality in subjects with type 2 diabetes i.e. increase in both IkappaB alpha and IkappaB beta protein, IkappaB alpha and IkappaB beta protein,

decrease in tumor necrosis factor alpha muscle content and an increase in insulin-stimulated glucose disposal [104].

9. Training significantly improved glucose tolerance in obese humans [105]. This may be benefit in control blood glucose concentration leading to prevention for patients diabetes type II.

10. Both moderate- and vigorous-intensity exercise training improved beta-cell function to the extent that the disposition index (DI) accurately reflects beta-cell function. Although through distinct mechanisms [106] were modeled from an intravenous glucose tolerance test. [DI = S(i) x AIRg (insulin sensitivity (S(i)), acute insulin response to glucose (AIRg)]

11. In diabetic rats, exendin-4 and exercise stimulate insulin receptor substrate (IRS)-2 expression [107, 108] through the activation of cAMP responding element binding protein in the islets [109]. This enhanced their insulin/insulin like growth factor-1 signaling. The potentiation of the signaling increased the expression of pancreas duodenum homeo-box-1, involved in beta-cell proliferation. In conclusion, exendin-4 and exercise equivalently improved glucose homeostasis due to the induction of IRS-2 in the islets of diabetic rats through a cAMP dependent common pathway.

12. Exercise training substantially reduces the exposure of islets to exogenous lipid, thereby providing a potential mechanism by which exercise can prevent islet beta-cell failure leading to diabetes type 2 [110].

13. Exercise may have beneficial effects via monocyte since monocyte peroxisome proliferator activated receptors gamma (PPARγ) activation has been linked to beneficial antidiabetic effects. This is supported by the association between exercise-induced upregulation of monocytic PPARγ-controlled genes and reverse cholesterol transport and anti-inflammatory effects. Thus, exercise-induced monocyte PPARγ activation may contribute to rationale for prescribing exercise to type 2 diabetes patients [111].

14. High-intensity progressive resistance training, in combination with moderate weight loss, effectively improved glycemic control in older patients with type 2 diabetes. This may result from increased muscle mass leading to increased glucose uptake [112].

6.3. Weight reduction

Swim training can effectively prevent body weight gain, adiposity and lipid disorders caused by leptin receptor deficiency, in part through activation of UCPs in adipose tissue and skeletal muscle [113]. The training also increased carnitine palmitoyl transferase (CPT I) activity and became less sensitive to inhibition by malonyl-CoA, reduced both total ceramide content. In addition, it improved capacity for mitochondrial FA uptake and oxidation leads not only to a reduction in muscle lipid content but also to change in the saturation status of lipids [114]. These may contribute to alleviating weight reduction for patients with diabetes type 2.

6.4. Normalization of blood lipid profiles

Decreases in total cholesterol, increases in HDL, oxidized LDL (oxLDL), leukocyte mRNA expression for PPARgamma which was reinforced by increased PPARgamma DNA-binding activity and gene expression were observed for the oxLDL scavenger receptor CD36 LXRalpha. Two LXRalpha-regulated genes involved in RCT, namely, ATP-binding cassette transporters A1 and GI (ABCA1 and ABCG1, respectively), were significantly up-regulated post-exercise [115].

6.5. Improved nitric oxide-mediated skeletal muscle blood flow

1. Exercise training improves endothelium-dependent vasodilator function, not only as a localised phenomenon in the contracting muscle group, but also as a systemic response when a relatively large mass of muscle is activated regularly during an exercise training program. Shear stress-mediated improvement in endothelial function provides one plausible explanation for the cardioprotective benefits of exercise training [116].

2. In addition to being a possible modulator of blood flow, nitric oxide (NO) from skeletal muscle regulates muscle contraction and metabolism. Recently, human data indicate that NO plays a role in muscle glucose uptake during exercise independently of blood flow. Exercise training in healthy individuals increased NO bioavailability through a variety of mechanisms including increased NOS enzyme expression and activity. This contributed to increased exercise capacity and cardiovascular protection. Exercise training with high cardiovascular risk can increase NO bioavailability and may represent an important mechanism by which exercise training takes benefit in the prevention [117].

6.6. Improvement of nervous system function

Progressive exercise training significantly decreases diabetes-associated neuropathic pain, including thermal hyperalgesia and mechanical allodynia. In rats, this protective effect is related to the increase of Hsp72, but not TNF-α and IL-6, expression in the spinal cord and peripheral nerves of STZ-induced diabetes. [118]

6.7. Improved oxidative stress

Acute exercise was reported to elevate Ox LDL, SOD and GSH-Px levels which are associated with in type 2 diabetic patients [119]. Exercise training including low-intensity exercise can increase antioxidant and decrease oxidant [72]

6.8. Prevention of microangiopathy

Mitochondrial oxidative capacity appears to be involved in the overall mechanism by which exercise prevents microangiopathy in rats with type 2 diabetes. Luminal capillary diameter of the diabetic group was significantly lower than that of the control group, succinic dehydrogenase (SDH) activity was significantly higher in the diabetic with exercise group than in the control and diabetic groups [120].

6.9. Improve metabolic control

Exercise training results in an increase in the oxidative capacity of skeletal muscle by up-regulating lipid oxidation and the expression of proteins involved in mitochondrial biogenesis. This decreased liver triacylglycerol content [121].

Acknowledgements

This study was supported by a grant from Thailand Research Fund (TRF). The authors appreciate Associate Professor Jongonnee Wattanapermpool for her excellent assistance with critical commentary and suggestions. The authors thank Assistant Professor Dr. Thongchai Pratipanawatr for his invaluable assistance with data acquisition. The authors also thank Ms Saovanee Luangaram for her excellent measurement of oxidative stress. The authors appreciate all patients who participated in this study.

This chapter was supported by Exercise and Sport Sciences Research and Development Group.

Author details

Naruemon Leelayuwat*

Address all correspondence to: naruemon@kku.ac.th

Department of Physiology, Faculty of Medicine, Khon Kaen University, Thailand

References

[1] http://www.swfhealthandwellness.com/alternative-exercises-3-02

[2] Berry TR, Chan CB, Bell RC, Walker J. Collective knowledge: using a consensus conference approach to develop recommendations for physical activity and nutrition programs for persons with type 2 diabetes. Frontiers in Endocrinol (Lausanne) 2012;3:161. doi: 10.3389/fendo.2012.00161. Epub 2012 Dec 11.

[3] Buse JB, Ginsberg HN, Bakris GL, Clark NG, Costa F, Eckel R, et al. Primary prevention of cardiovascular diseases in people with diabetes mellitus: a scientific statement from the American Heart Association and the American Diabetes Association, Circulation 2007;115:114-126.

[4] http://ww1.prweb.com/prfiles/2011/12/19/10360439/Yoga%20Warrior%20Pose %202.jpg (accessed 22 February 2013).

[5]   http://kateasana.wordpress.com/2012/07/02/announcing-the-great-108-challenge-and-august-yoga-in-the-park/ (accessed 25 February 2013)

[6]   http://yoga.about.com/od/beginningyoga/a/whatisyoga.htm (accessed 25 February 2013)

[7]   Madanmohan, Bhavanani AB, Dayanidy G, Sanjay Z, Basavaraddi IV. Effect of yoga therapy on reaction time, biochemical parameters and wellness score of peri and post-menopausal diabetic patients. International journal of yoga 2012;5(1):10-15. doi: 10.4103/0973-6131.91696.

[8]   Kyizom T, Singh S, Singh KP, Tandon OP, Kumar R. Effect of pranayama & yoga-asana on cognitive brain functions in type 2 diabetes-P3 event related evoked potential (ERP). The Indian journal of medical research 2010;131:636-640.

[9]   Hegde SV, Adhikari P, Kotian S, Pinto VJ, D'Souza S, D'Souza V. Effect of 3-month yoga on oxidative stress in type 2 diabetes with or without complications: a controlled clinical trial. Diabetes Care. 2011;34(10):2208-2210. doi: 10.2337/dc10-2430. Epub 2011 Aug 11.

[10] Malhotra V, Singh S, Tandon OP, Madhu SV, Prasad A, Sharma SB. Effect of Yoga asanas on nerve conduction in type 2 diabetes. Indian journal of physiology and pharmacology 2002;46(3):298-306.

[11] Kosuri M, Sridhar GR. Yoga practice in diabetes improves physical and psychological outcomes. Metabolic syndrome and related disorders 2009;7(6):515-517. doi: 10.1089/met.2009.0011.

[12] Yang K, Bernardo LM, Sereika SM, Conroy MB, Balk J, Burke LE. Utilization of 3-month yoga program for adults at high risk for type 2 diabetes: a pilot study. Evidence-based complementary and alternative medicine 2011;2011:257891. doi: 10.1093/ecam/nep117. Epub 2011 Jan 9.

[13] Amita S, Prabhakar S, Manoj I, Harminder S, Pavan T. Effect of yoga-nidra on blood glucose level in diabetic patients. Indian journal of physiology and pharmacology 2009;53(1):97-101.

[14] Malhotra V, Singh S, Singh KP, Gupta P, Sharma SB, Madhu SV, Tandon OP. Study of yoga asanas in assessment of pulmonary function in NIDDM patients. Indian journal of physiology and pharmacology 2002;46(3):313-320.

[15] Jyotsna VP, Joshi A, Ambekar S, Kumar N, Dhawan A, Sreenivas V. Comprehensive yogic breathing program improves quality of life in patients with diabetes. Indian journal of endocrinology and metabolism 2012;16(3):423-428. doi: 10.4103/2230-8210.95692.

[16] http://www.fitnessrxwomen.com/training/alternative-training/yoga/ (accessed 25 February 2013)

[17] "Bikram's Yoga College of India". Bikramyoga.com. Retrieved 2011-12-28.

[18] Corporate registration for "Bikram Choudhury Yoga, Inc." Number: C2288343

[19] Farrell, M. (September 3, 2009). "Bikram Yoga's New Twists". Forbes.com.

[20] Wilson, Cynthia. "Different types of yoga and their benefits". Womenio. Retrieved 26 September 2012.

[21] http://www.readersdigest.com.au/alternative-exercise-ideas (accessed 25 February 2013)

[22] http://universal-taichichuan.com/restoring-your-qi-with-tai-chi/ (accessed 25 February 2013)

[23] Liu X, Miller YD, Burton NW, Chang JH, Brown WJ. The effect of Tai Chi on health-related quality of life in people with elevated blood glucose or diabetes: a randomized controlled trial. Quality of life research 2012 Nov 10. [Epub ahead of print]

[24] Hung JW, Liou CW, Wang PW, Yeh SH, Lin LW, Lo SK, Tsai FM. Effect of 12-week tai chi chuan exercise on peripheral nerve modulation in patients with type 2 diabetes mellitus. Journal of rehabilitation medicine 2009;41(11):924-929. doi: 10.2340/16501977-0445.

[25] Lam P, Dennis SM, Diamond TH, Zwar N. Improving glycaemic and BP control in type 2 diabetes. The effectiveness of tai chi. Australian family physician 2008;37(10): 884-887.

[26] Chen SC, Ueng KC, Lee SH, Sun KT, Lee MC. Effect of t'ai chi exercise on biochemical profiles and oxidative stress indicators in obese patients with type 2diabetes. Journal of alternative and complementary medicine (New York, N.Y.) 2010;16(11): 1153-1159. doi: 10.1089/acm.2009.0560. Epub 2010 Oct 25.

[27] Field T. Tai Chi research review. Complementary therapies in clinical practice 2011 Aug;17(3):141-6. doi: 10.1016/j.ctcp.2010.10.002. Epub 2010 Oct 24.

[28] Song R, Ahn S, Roberts BL, Lee EO, Ahn YH. Adhering to a t'ai chi program to improve glucose control and quality of life for individuals with type 2 diabetes. Journal of alternative and complementary medicine (New York, N.Y.) 2009;15(6):627-632. doi: 10.1089/acm.2008.0330.

[29] Lee MS, Choi TY, Lim HJ, Ernst E. Tai chi for management of type 2 diabetes mellitus: A systematic review. Chinese journal of integrative medicine 2011 Jul 30. [Epub ahead of print]

[30] http://www.spirityogaonline.com/massage.html (accessed 25 February 2013)

[31] http://www.marycatherinestarr.com/2/post/2011/03/life-changing-discovery-thai-yoga-massage.html (accessed 25 February 2013)

[32] Buranruk O, La Grow S, Ladawan S, Makarawate P, Suwanich T, and Leelayuwat N. Thai Yoga as an Appropriate Alternative Physical Activity for Older Adults. Journal of Complementary and Integrative Medicine 2010;7:1-14.

[33] Puengsuwan P, Promdee K, Sruttabul W, Na Nagara R, Leelayuwat N. Effectiveness of Thai Wand Exercise training on health-related quality of life in sedentary older adults. Chulalongorn Medicine Journal 2008;52:120-122.

[34] http://www.kendimiz.com/tag/martial-arts-boxing-chaiya/ (accessed 25 February 2013)

[35] http://www.superprosamui.com/muay-thai/muay-thai-martial-arts.html (accessed 25 February 2013)

[36] http://en.wikipedia.org/wiki/Chinese_martial_arts (accessed 23 February 2013)

[37] http://en.wikipedia.org/wiki/Martial_arts (accessed 23 February 2013)

[38] http://en.wikipedia.org/wiki/Taekwondo (accessed 24 February 2013)

[39] http://www.eonline.com/news/355888/melissa-rycroft-released-from-hospital-after-dancing-with-the-stars-head-injury (accessed 24 February 2013)

[40] http://www.colourbox.com/vector/silhouettes-of-the-pairs-dancing-ballroom-dances-tango-vector-4335705 (accessed 24 February 2013)

[41] Hogg J, Diaz A, Del Cid M, Mueller C, Lipman EG, Cheruvu S, Chiu YL, Vogiatzi M, Nimkarn S. An after-school dance and lifestyle education program reduces risk factors for heart disease and diabetes in elementary school children. Journal of pediatric endocrinology & metabolism 2012;25(5-6):509-516.

[42] Murrock CJ, Higgins PA, Killion C. Dance and peer support to improve diabetes outcomes in African American women. Diabetes Education 2009;35(6):995-1003. doi: 10.1177/0145721709343322. Epub 2009 Sep 23.

[43] Tudor-Locke C, Schuna JM Jr. Steps to preventing type 2 diabetes: exercise, walk more, or sit less? Frontiers Endocrinology (Lausanne). 2012;3:142. doi: 10.3389/fendo.2012.00142. Epub 2012 Nov 19.

[44] http://www.mayoclinic.com/health/walking/SM00062_D (accessed 24 February 2013)

[45] http://walking.about.com/od/workouts/a/Brisk-Walking.htm (accessed 24 February 2013)

[46] http://www.worcestershiretouristguides.com/Articles/Article_168.asp (accessed 24 February 2013)

[47] http://www.realbuzz.com/articles/alternative-exercise-activities-gb-en/ (accessed 23 February 2013)

[48] http://www.telegraph.co.uk/sport/olympics/sailing/9463023/Saskia-Clark-and-Hannah-Mills-on-target-for-sailing-Olympic-gold.html (accessed 24 February 2013)

[49] http://www.horse-insurance.co.uk/blog/news/pioneering-new-therapy-offers-hope-for-spinal-injuries/attachment/horse-riding-spinal-injury/ (accessed 24 February 2013)

[50] http://www.globaltravelmate.com/asia/thailand/phuket/phuket-to-do/590-phuket-horse-riding-club.html (accessed 26 February 2013)

[51] Hosaka Y, Nagasaki M, Bajotto G, Shinomiya Y, Ozawa T, Sato Y. Effects of daily mechanical horseback riding on insulin sensitivity and resting metabolism in middle-aged type 2 diabetes mellitus patients. Nagoya journal of medical science 2010 Aug; 72(3-4):129-137.

[52] Kubota M, Nagasaki M, Tokudome M, Shinomiya Y, Ozawa T, Sato Y. Mechanical horseback riding improves insulin sensitivity in elder diabetic patients. Diabetes Research and Clinical Practice 2006;71(2):124-130. Epub 2005 Aug 18.

[53] http://californiaoutdoorsqas.com/2009/04/02/whereas-the-year-round-trout-fishing/ (accessed 26 February 2013)

[54] http://www.fitsugar.com/Back-Basics-Walking-Forward-Lunge-174913 (accessed 25 February 2013)

[55] http://www.chatelaine.com/tag/burn-calories/ (accessed 25 February 2013) (accessed 25 February 2013)

[56] http://www.huntingdonpeople.co.uk/sport/Fit-Huntingdon-s-Great-Outdoors/story-4529771-detail/story.html (accessed 26 February 2013)

[57] http://surfandlong.blogspot.com/ (accessed 25 February 2013)

[58] http://www.gocardiotennis.net/ (accessed 25 February 2013)

[59] http://sicefamily.blogspot.com/2012/03/make-change-learning-to-love-exercise.html (accessed 25 February 2013)

[60] http://images.yourdictionary.com/housework (accessed 25 February 2013)

[61] http://www.rodale.com/burn-calories-cleaning-house (accessed 25 February 2013)

[62] http://www.alexandertechnique.com/photos/ (accessed 25 February 2013)

[63] Woodman, J.P.; Moore, N.R. (2012). "Evidence for the effectiveness of Alexander Technique lessons in medical and health-related conditions: a systematic review". International Journal of Clinical Practice 66(1): 98–112. doi:10.1111/j.1742-1241.2011.02817.x. PMID 22171910

[64] http://wakeup-feldenkrais.blogspot.com/2007/03/new-version-what-is-feldenkrais-method.html (accessed 25 February 2013)

[65] http://en.wikipedia.org/wiki/Feldenkrais_Method (accessed 26 February 2013)

[66] Strauch R. An overview of the Feldenkrais Method. retrieved 14 May 2008

[67] http://www.muscle-fitness-tips.net/pilates-exercises.html (accessed 26 February 2013)

[68] http://pilates.about.com/od/intermediateadvexercises/ss/Side-Stretch-Pilates-Exercises_4.htm (accessed 26 February 2013)

[69] http://www.glamour.com/health-fitness/blogs/vitamin-g/2013/02/5-pilates-moves-thatll-blast-y.html (accessed 26 February 2013)

[70] http://en.wikipedia.org/wiki/Pilates (accessed 26 February 2013)

[71] Mayo Clinic Staff (2012). "Pilates for Beginners: Explore the Core of Pilates". Mayo Clinic. Retrieved 2012-11-04

[72] Leelayuwat N, Tunkumnerdthai O, Donsom M, Punyaek N, Manimanakorn A, KukongviriyapanU, Kukongviriyapan V. An alternative exercise and its beneficial effects on glycaemic control and oxidative stress in subjects with type 2 diabetes. Diabetes Research and Clinical Practice 2008;82:e5–e8.

[73] Jwing-Ming Y. (2002). Swinging the Arms or Bai Bi. from. http://dactrung.net/truyen/noidung.aspx?BaiID=zlz3sRQzM57p%2Bhp8g9wOUg%3D%3D (accessed 18 Jun, 2008).

[74] Matthews MR, Hosker JP, Rudenski AS, Naylor BA, Treacher DF, Turner RC, Homeostasis model assessment: insulin resistance and beta-cell function from fasting plasma glucose and insulin concentrations in man, Diabetologia 28 (1985) 412-419.

[75] Jeng C, Chang WY, Chen SR, Tseng IJ. Effects of arm exercise on serum glucose response in type 2 DM patients. The journal of nursing research 2002;10:187-194.

[76] Maiorana A, O'Driscoll G, Goodman C, Taylor R, Green D. Combined aerobic and resistance exercise improves glycemic control and fitness in type 2 diabetes. Diabetes Research and Clinical Practice 2002;56:115-123.

[77] Tsujiuchi T, Kumano H, Yoshiuchi K, He D, Tsujiuchi Y, Kuboki T et al. The effect of Qi-gong relaxation exercise on the control of type 2 diabetes mellitus: a randomized controlled trial. Diabetes Care 2002;25: 241-242.

[78] Stratton IM, Adler AI, Neil HAW, Matthews DR, Manley SE, Cull CA et al. on behalf of the UK Prospective Diabetes Study Group. Association of glycaemia with macrovascular and microvascular complications of type 2 diabetes (UKPDS 35): prospective observational study. BMJ 2000;321:405-412.

[79] Ding Y, Kantarci A, Hasturk H, Trackman PC, Malabanan A, Van Dyke TE. Activation of RAGE induces elevated O^{2-} generation by mononuclear phagocytes in diabetes, Journal of leukocyte biology 2007;81:520-527.

[80] Ciuchi E, Odetti P, Prando R, Relationship between glutathione and sorbitol concentrations in erythrocytes from diabetic patients. Metabolism 1996;45:611-613.

[81] Sathiyapriya V, Selvaraj N, Nandeesha H, Bobby Z, Agrawal A, Pavithran P. Enhanced glycation of hemoglobin and plasma proteins is associated with increased lipid peroxide levels in non-diabetic hypertensive subjects. Archives of Medical Research 2007;38:822-826.

[82] Yamagishi S, Imaizumi T. Diabetic vascular complications: pathophysiology, biochemical basis and potential therapeutic strategy. Current Pharmaceutical Design 2005;11: 2279-2299.

[83] Kaczor JJ, Hall JE, Payne E, Tarnopolsky MA. Low intensity training decreases markers of oxidative stress in skeletal muscle of mdx mice. Free Radical Biology & Medicine 2007;43:145-154.

[84] Covas MI, Elosua R, Fitó M, Alcantara M, Coca L, Marrugat J. Relationship between physical activity and oxidative stress biomarkers in women. Medicine & Science in Sports & Exercise 2002;34:814-819.

[85] Heitcamp HC, Wegler S, Brehme U, Heinle H. Effect of an 8-week endurance training program on markers of antioxidant capacity in women. The Journal of Sports Medicine and Physical Fitness 2008;48:113-119.

[86] Moien-Afshari F, Ghosh S, Khazaei M, Kieffer TJ, Brownsey RW, Laher I. Exercise restores endothelial function independently of weight loss or hyperglycaemic status in db/db mice. Diabetologia 2008 Apr 25. [Epub ahead of print]

[87] Zierath, Juleen R. Invited Review: Exercise training-induced changes in insulin signaling in skeletal muscle. J Appl Physiol 93: 773–781, 2002;10.1152/japplphysiol. 00126.2002.

[88] Goodyear LJ, Chang PY, Sherwood DJ, Dufresne SD, Moller DE. Effects of exercise and insulin on mitogen-activated protein kinase signaling pathways in rat skeletal muscle. Am J Physiol. 1996 Aug;271(2 Pt 1):E403-8.

[89] Lee H, Chang H, Park JY, Kim SY, Choi KM, Song W. Exercise training improves basal blood glucose metabolism with no changes of cytosolic inhibitor B kinase or c-Jun N-terminal kinase activation in skeletal muscle of Otsuka Long-Evans Tokushima fatty rats. Exp Physiol. 2011 Jul;96(7):689-98. doi: 10.1113/expphysiol.2011.057737. Epub 2011 Apr 28.

[90] Castaneda F, Layne JE, Castaneda C. Skeletal muscle sodium glucose co-transporters in older adults with type 2 diabetes undergoing resistance training. Int J Med Sci. 2006;3(3):84-91. Epub 2006 May 17.

[91] Christ-Roberts CY, Pratipanawatr T, Pratipanawatr W, Berria R, Belfort R, Kashyap S, Mandarino LJ. Exercise training increases glycogen synthase activity and GLUT4

expression but not insulin signaling in overweight nondiabetic and type 2 diabetic subjects. Metabolism. 2004 Sep;53(9):1233-42.

[92] Thyfault JP, Cree MG, Zheng D, Zwetsloot JJ, Tapscott EB, Koves TR, Ilkayeva O, Wolfe RR, Muoio DM, Dohm GL. Contraction of insulin-resistant muscle normalizes insulin action in association with increased mitochondrial activity and fatty acid catabolism. Am J Physiol Cell Physiol. 2007 Feb;292(2):C729-39. Epub 2006 Oct 18.

[93] Hawley JA. Exercise as a therapeutic intervention for the prevention and treatment of insulin resistance. Diabetes Metab Res Rev. 2004 Sep-Oct;20(5):383-93.

[94] Ryder JW, Chibalin AV, Zierath JR. Intracellular mechanisms underlying increases in glucose uptake in response to insulin or exercise in skeletal muscle. Acta Physiol Scand. 2001 Mar;171(3):249-57.

[95] Frøsig C, Richter EA. Improved insulin sensitivity after exercise: focus on insulin signaling. Obesity (Silver Spring). 2009 Dec;17 Suppl 3:S15-20. doi: 10.1038/oby.2009.383.

[96] Matos A, Ropelle ER, Pauli JR, Frederico MJ, de Pinho RA, Velloso LA, De Souza CT. Acute exercise reverses TRB3 expression in the skeletal muscle and ameliorates whole body insulin sensitivity in diabetic mice. Acta Physiol (Oxf). 2010 Jan;198(1): 61-9. doi: 10.1111/j.1748-1716.2009.02031.x. Epub 2009 Aug 12.

[97] Costford SR, Bajpeyi S, Pasarica M, Albarado DC, Thomas SC, Xie H, Church TS, Jubrias SA, Conley KE, Smith SR. Skeletal muscle NAMPT is induced by exercise in humans. Am J Physiol Endocrinol Metab. 2010 Jan;298(1):E117-26. doi: 10.1152/ajpendo.00318.2009. Epub 2009 Nov 3.

[98] Manabe Y, Gollisch KS, Holton L, Kim YB, Brandauer J, Fujii NL, Hirshman MF, Goodyear LJ. Exercise training-induced adaptations associated with increases in skeletal muscle glycogen content. FEBS J. 2013 Feb;280(3):916-26. doi: 10.1111/febs.12085. Epub 2013 Jan 7.

[99] Perseghin G, Price TB, Petersen KF, Roden M, Cline GW, Gerow K, Rothman DL, Shulman GI. Increased glucose transport-phosphorylation and muscle glycogen synthesis after exercise training in insulin-resistant subjects. N Engl J Med. 1996 Oct 31;335(18):1357-62.

[100] Kiilerich K, Gudmundsson M, Birk JB, Lundby C, Taudorf S, Plomgaard P, Saltin B, Pedersen PA, Wojtaszewski JF, Pilegaard HDiabetes. Low muscle glycogen and elevated plasma free fatty acid modify but do not prevent exercise-induced PDH activation in human skeletal muscle. 2010 Jan;59(1):26-32. doi: 10.2337/db09-1032. Epub 2009 Oct 15.

[101] Wang Y, Simar D, Fiatarone Singh MA. Adaptations to exercise training within skeletal muscle in adults with type 2 diabetes or impaired glucose tolerance: a systematic review. Diabetes Metab Res Rev. 2009 Jan;25(1):13-40. doi: 10.1002/dmrr.928.

[102] Hawley JA, Lessard SJ. Exercise training-induced improvements in insulin action. Acta Physiol (Oxf). 2008 Jan;192(1):127-35. doi: 10.1111/j.1748-1716.2007.01783.x.

[103] Cao S, Li B, Yi X, Chang B, Zhu B, Lian Z, Zhang Z, Zhao G, Liu H, Zhang H. Effects of exercise on AMPK signaling and downstream components to PI3K in rat with type 2 diabetes. PLoS One. 2012;7(12):e51709. doi: 10.1371/journal.pone.0051709. Epub 2012 Dec 13.

[104] Sriwijitkamol A, Christ-Roberts C, Berria R, Eagan P, Pratipanawatr T, DeFronzo RA, Mandarino LJ, Musi N. Reduced skeletal muscle inhibitor of kappaB beta content is associated with insulin resistance in subjects with type 2 diabetes: reversal by exercise training. Diabetes. 2006 Mar;55(3):760-7.

[105] Bruce CR, Thrush AB, Mertz VA, Bezaire V, Chabowski A, Heigenhauser GJ, Dyck DJ. Endurance training in obese humans improves glucose tolerance and mitochondrial fatty acid oxidation and alters muscle lipid content. Am J Physiol Endocrinol Metab. 2006 Jul;291(1):E99-E107. Epub 2006 Feb 7.

[106] Slentz CA, Tanner CJ, Bateman LA, Durheim MT, Huffman KM, Houmard JA, Kraus WE. Effects of exercise training intensity on pancreatic beta-cell function. Diabetes Care. 2009 Oct;32(10):1807-11. doi: 10.2337/dc09-0032. Epub 2009 Jul 10.

[107] Park S, Hong SM, Sung SR. Exendin-4 and exercise promotes beta-cell function and mass through IRS2 induction in islets of diabetic rats. Life Sci. 2008 Feb 27;82(9-10): 503-11. doi: 10.1016/j.lfs.2007.12.018. Epub 2007 Dec 31.

[108] Park S, Hong SM, Lee JE, Sung SR. Moreover, exercise improves glucose homeostasis that has been impaired by a high-fat diet by potentiating pancreatic beta-cell function and mass through IRS2 in diabetic rats. J Appl Physiol. 2007 Nov;103(5):1764-71. Epub 2007 Aug 30.

[109] Choi SB, Jang JS, Park S. Estrogen and exercise may enhance beta-cell function and mass via insulin receptor substrate 2 induction in ovariectomized diabetic rats. Endocrinology. 2005 Nov;146(11):4786-94. Epub 2005 Jul 21.

[110] Lamontagne J, Masiello P, Marcil M, Delghingaro-Augusto V, Burelle Y, Prentki M, Nolan CJ. Circulating lipids are lowered but pancreatic islet lipid metabolism and insulin secretion are unaltered in exercise-trained female rats. Appl Physiol Nutr Metab. 2007 Apr;32(2):241-8.

[111] Thomas AW, Davies NA, Moir H, Watkeys L, Ruffino JS, Isa SA, Butcher LR, Hughes MG, Morris K, Webb R. Exercise-associated generation of PPARγ ligands activates PPARγ signaling events and upregulates genes related to lipid metabolism. J Appl Physiol. 2012 Mar;112(5):806-15. doi: 10.1152/japplphysiol.00864.2011. Epub 2011 Dec 15.

[112]   Dunstan DW, Daly RM, Owen N, Jolley D, De Courten M, Shaw J, Zimmet P. High-intensity resistance training improves glycemic control in older patients with type 2 diabetes. Diabetes Care. 2002 Oct;25(10):1729-36.

[113]   Oh KS, Kim EY, Yoon M, Lee CM. Swim training improves leptin receptor deficiency-induced obesity and lipid disorder by activating uncoupling proteins. Exp Mol Med. 2007 Jun 30;39(3):385-94.

[114]   Bruce CR, Thrush AB, Mertz VA, Bezaire V, Chabowski A, Heigenhauser GJ, Dyck DJ. Endurance training in obese humans improves glucose tolerance and mitochondrial fatty acid oxidation and alters muscle lipid content. Am J Physiol Endocrinol Metab. 2006 Jul;291(1):E99-E107. Epub 2006 Feb 7.

[115]   Butcher LR, Thomas A, Backx K, Roberts A, Webb R, Morris K. Low-intensity exercise exerts beneficial effects on plasma lipids via PPARgamma. Med Sci Sports Exerc. 2008 Jul;40(7):1263-70. doi: 10.1249/MSS.0b013e31816c091d.

[116]   J Appl Physiol. 2004 Nov;97(5):1823-9. Epub 2004 Jun 18. Exercise alters the profile of phospholipid molecular species in rat skeletal muscle. Mitchell TW, Turner N, Hulbert AJ, Else PL, Hawley JA, Lee JS, Bruce CR, Blanksby SJ.

[117]   Kingwell BA. Nitric oxide-mediated metabolic regulation during exercise: effects of training in health and cardiovascular disease. FASEB J. 2000 Sep;14(12):1685-96.

[118]   Chen YW, Hsieh PL, Chen YC, Hung CH, Cheng JT. Physical exercise induces excess hsp72 expression and delays the development of hyperalgesia and allodynia in painful diabetic neuropathy rats. Anesth Analg. 2013 Feb;116(2):482-90. doi: 10.1213/ANE. 0b013e318274e4a0. Epub 2013 Jan 9.

[119]   Vojnosanit Pregl. 2009 Jun;66(6):459-64. Clinical evaluation of oxidative stress in patients with diabetes mellitus type II -- impact of acute exercise. Kostić N, Caparević Z, Marina D, Ilić S, Radojković J, Cosić Z, Bakić-Celić V.

[120]   Morifuji T, Murakami S, Fujita N, Kondo H, Fujino H. Exercise training prevents decrease in luminal capillary diameter of skeletal muscles in rats with type 2 diabetes. Scientific World Journal. 2012;2012:645891. doi: 10.1100/2012/645891. Epub 2012 Aug 13.

[121]   Lessard SJ, Rivas DA, Chen ZP, Bonen A, Febbraio MA, Reeder DW, Kemp BE, Yaspelkis BB 3rd, Hawley JA. Tissue-specific effects of rosiglitazone and exercise in the treatment of lipid-induced insulin resistance. Diabetes. 2007 Jul;56(7):1856-64. Epub 2007 Apr 17.

Chapter 9

Psychodiabetic Kit and Its Application in Clinical Practice and Research

Andrzej Kokoszka, Aleksandra Jodko-Modlińska,
Marcin Obrębski, Joanna Ostasz-Ważny and
Rafał Radzio

Additional information is available at the end of the chapter

1. Introduction

A patient-centered approach is recommended for the management of diabetes type 2 by the American Diabetes Association and the European Association for the Study of Diabetes [1] "These recommendations should be considered within the context of the needs, preferences, and tolerances of each patient; individualization of treatment is the cornerstone of success. (…). The implementation of these guidelines will require thoughtful clinicians to integrate current evidence with other constraints and imperatives in the context of patient-specific factors" [1. p. 1364]. It includes taking into consideration the variable and progressive nature of type 2 diabetes, the specific role of each drug, the patient and disease factors that drive clinical decision making, and the constraints imposed by age and comorbidity. This implies diagnosis of psychosocial factors in regular medical practice. This is justified by sterling data indicating that psychosocial factors have meaningful impact on the management of diabetes. There is extensive literature suggesting that the patient's mental state has a profound impact on adherence to medical recommendations [2] and influences the course of the disease. Major diabetic problems are more widespread among patients with clinical depression, than those with subthreshold depression [3]. On the other hand, depression is more common among people with diabetes than in general population [4], and even in its subclinical form, it increases the risk of complications [5]. Research points to a link between the intensity of diabetes treatment and the occurrence of depressive mood [2]. It also indicates that the course of the disease affects the patient's ability to cope with stressful situations [6] and sense of control over the disease [7]. Many conducted studies reveal the importance of psychosocial factors in diabetes self-care. Diabetes-related emotional distress is connected with difficulties with diabetes self-management and poor glycemic control [8]. Self-efficacy and problem solving were associated with self-management behaviors like healthy eating and physical activity [9]. It is known that patients understand the importance of diabetes management and the consequences of bad metabolic control. Their poor control results not from a lack of knowledge but on the way diabetes is prioritised in their lives [10]. There is evidence that diabetes management is strongly influenced by psychosocial factors [11]. This implies the necessity of inclusion of diagnosis of psychological and psychotherapeutic factors during a routine visit of patients with diabetes. Team approach in this management, including diabetologist, nurse, psychologist, educator, and social worker is optimal. However, in many countries significant rates of outpatient clinics can offer their patients therapeutic interventions made only by doctors and the nurses. Working in such setting they need diagnositic and therapeutic tools helpful in management of psychosocial problems related with diabetes. However, the number of tolls that are useful in such conditions is limited. The computerized assessment tool "Monitoring of Individual Needs in persons with Diabetes" (MIND) [12,13] includes World Health Organization's Five Well-being index (WHO-5) [14,15], Problem Areas In Diabetes (PAID) [16-18], life events and patient's agenda, can be used for diagnosis of psychosocial factors connected to diabetes management. Analysis of data from the cross-national Diabetes Attitudes Wishes and Needs (DAWN) MIND study, conducted in 8 countries, also in our center in Poland, confirmed that "MIND" computer procedure is feasible as a part of ongoing diabetes care and helps to identify unmet psychosocial needs in diabetes patients. However it does not help in psychotherapeutic diagnosis that is needed for the basic psychotherapeutic interventions that can be made by doctors during a regular visit[12,13]. The psychodiabetic KIT was elaborated in response to such needs. The analysis of literature in MEDLINE and PUBMED indicates that there are no concise comprehensive diagnostic tools for supporting psychotherapeutic diagnosis during the regular medical visit of patients with diabetes and there are no simple psychotherapeutic strategies of interventions in such a setting. Psychodiabetic KIT supports a diagnosis of coping styles, perception of self-influence on diabetes course and a more reliable diagnosis of depression and anxiety, than the one WHO-5 and PAID used as screening tools for depression. In this chapter we describe: a theoretical rationale of the Psychodiabetic Kit, three tools that it comprises together with "The Practical Schema of Psychotherapeutic Management within a Regular Medical Visit" as well as a review of research confirming its usefulness both in research and clinical practice.

2. Rationale of psychodiabetic KIT

Improvement of patients' adherence to the optimum management of diabetes may be considered as the target of psychotherapeutic interventions during medical visits, when education about the diabetes is not efficient. The theoretical framework of psychotherapeutic diagnosis and interventions should be easy to understand for both therapists and patients. It was presumed that due to the common time constrains the diagnostic tools should:

1. be brief

2. compromise goals of enhancing psychological thinking and psychometric proprieties

3. rather support the clinical psychological diagnosis, than replace it

4.   promote psychological understanding both of the patient and of the therapist

5.   integrate the psychological diagnosis and interventions with the regular clinical management

Eventually the concept of coping with stress was chosen as theoretical background for the diagnosis. Whereas the practical interventions following the recommendations of the International Diabetes Association [19] are based on philosophy of empowerment, and rule self-management [19,20], that applies elements of behavioral therapy.

The concept of coping with stress related with diabetes and perception of self-influence on the diabetes course

Coping is defined as 'constantly changing cognitive and behavioral efforts to manage specific external and/or internal demands that are appraised as taxing or exceeding the resources of the person [21]. Coping is an adaptation activity that involves effort and aims to diminish the physical, emotional, and psychological burden linked to stressful life events [22]. However, the outcome of the coping process can also be maladaptation. The dispositional traits that influence how stressful events are assessed and that consequently determine the strategies a person uses to manage or address a stressor, may be described as coping strategies. Endler and Parker [23] offered simple classification of coping styles: task-oriented, emotion-oriented and avoidance-oriented. Patients utilizing an emotion- oriented strategy try to process reactions to stressor(s) by acting and thinking and in this scenario the person is focused on the emotion evoked by the stressor; overall, efforts are directed at altering the emotional responses. Patients who use a task-oriented strategy believe that they can prevail the situation caused by their disease or that they can adapt their resources to manage the situation, which often involves taking direct action to alter the situation itself. An avoidance-oriented coping style includes strategies such as avoiding a situation, denying its existence, or losing hope, via conscious and/or unconscious mechanisms; when using this coping style, the person also uses indirect efforts to adjust to stressors by distancing them, evading the problem, or engaging in unrelated activities to reduce feelings of stress. In addition to emotion-, task-, and avoidance-orientated, "the best solution oriented coping" style has been described [24]. When engaging in the 'identifying the best solution' coping style, the person actively searches for the most effective solutions, taking into account that they may be more "expensive" and risky than the standard ones. The classification of coping styles into just four main categories simplifies the understanding of these behaviors for both doctors and their patients. The concept of stress introduced by Seyle [25,26] is commonly known, unlike its most important developments dealing with the intensity of reactions to stressful events, that depends on [27] :

1.   How the challenge is evaluated, what's its meaning for the individual

2.   Which coping style is used

3.   What the level of social support is

Analysis of literature reveals a close relationship between an individual's overall psychological disposition and the cognitive and emotional aspects of their illness-coping strategies, which indirectly affect health-seeking behaviors [28]. According to the goodness of fit hypothesis, the effectiveness of problem- versus emotion-focused coping is moderated by appraisal of control over the stressful event [21,29]. The application of a problem-oriented coping style requires a feeling of control over the stressor, while in situations where there is an actual or perceived lack of control, an emotion-oriented or avoidance oriented coping style is applied. This concept has received some empirical support in a study involving patients with type 2 diabetes mellitus (T2DM) [30].

Indeed, among the variety of psychological factors described, the coping style and the perception of control over the disease course seem to have an important effect on outcomes in patients with diabetes [31,32]. Thus it is also likely that, in terms of coping strategies used to deal with diabetes, the individual's appraisal of illness as controllable or uncontrollable plays a role in the choice of strategy and therefore, ultimately, also in illness-associated outcomes.

In long-term progressive diseases, the concept of control is misleading because, in the majority of cases, even total adherence to the recommended treatment regimen can not guarantee restraining of either disease progress or recurrence of acute symptoms [7]. Perception of self-influence on a disease course can be defined as the extent of belief about one's own abilities to shape the disease course. It was formulated in response to data indicating that the coping style applied in response to a particular stressor is dependent on the perceived degree of control over that stressor [7]. As such, the concept of perceived self-influence on the disease course may be a more appropriate notion than control, when considering long-term progressive diseases, as even with chronic diseases, adherence to the recommended treatment and management plan can modify the disease course. Self influence also differs from perceived self-efficacy, which is defined as beliefs about the capabilities to produce designated levels of performance that exercise influence over events that affect lives. More specifically, self-efficacy beliefs determine how people feel, think, behave and motivate themselves [28], while perception of self-influence is related to disease management and is therefore more precise. Indeed, perceived control of diabetes was found to be a significant predictor of engagement in diabetes-specific health behaviors and positive perception of quality of life [31,32].

2.1. Depression and anxiety

Research analysis points to a high prevalence of depressive symptoms in a population of patients with diabetes [4,33]. Depression and its subclinical forms are connected to a negative course of diabetes. Depression is linked with poorer glicemic control [34]. Research confirms higher mortality in those groups of patients, in which major or moderate depression was diagnosed, when compared to a group in which depression was not found [35]. Moreover, patients reporting higher intensity of depressive symptoms are less willing to talk to their doctor about self-care [36]. Authors of the recent study, point that doctors need to be careful for depressive symptoms in their patients, and suggests the usefulness of brief diagnostic tools that may be used during a routine visit.

A higher prevalence of anxiety disorders and significant intensity of anxiety symptoms can also be observed among patients with diabetes [37,38]. The occurrence of those symptoms is connected to a poorer quality of life in diabetes patients [39]. The referred studies justify the purposefulness of evaluating depression and anxiety in patients with diabetes.

2.2. Description of the psychodiabetic KIT

Psychodiabetic KIT is a concise method of psychotherapeutic diagnosis and interventions aiming at improving the patient's adherence to therapeutic regimen. It was comprehensively described in a series of manuals [40-44] widely distributed among Polish diabetologists. Its application was discussed during many workshops. The Psychodiabetic Kit consists of:

1. Brief Methods of Evaluating Coping with Disease;

2. Brief Measure to Assess Perception of Self-Influence on the Disease Course: Version for Diabetes;

3. Brief Self-Rating Scale of Depression and Anxiety;

4. The Practical Schema of Psychotherapeutic Management within a Regular Medical Visit

The Brief Method of Evaluating Coping with Disease (BMECD; published in the appendix) [24] was created to assess the main four coping styles factors, which were mentioned above. This questionnaire consists of four questions with a choice of four behaviors. Each response relates to one of four distinguished coping styles related to aspects of life that are important for patients with diabetes (interpersonal, social, economic, and health related matters). The four BMECD questions are an outcome of a focus group interview with patients with T2DM who, in the opinion of their doctors, had developed either adaptive or maladaptive styles in order to cope with their disease. Data from the focus group were used by psychology students working on their Masters theses to generate 16 questions that related to typical methods of dealing with stressful situations according to each of the four main established coping styles. These 16 questions were correlated with the scores of the Coping Inventory for Stressful Situations (CISS) [45], the choice of the final four items was based on these results and on the opinion of two experienced clinical psychologists from the Medical University of Warsaw. Due to clinical observations indicating gender difficulties in perception and interpretation of some examples used in the questionnaire, which resulted in the reliability not being as satisfying as expected, the final version of BMECD [6] was elaborated. The changes included the descriptions of stressful situations adjusted to gender and to Polish language spelling by creating separate versions for males and females, and to making the test easier to read. The gender adjusted version has a relatively good reliability, as for an only four item questionnaire, designed for screening for maladaptive coping and as for an educational tool. Cronbach's alpha= 0.67 for avoidance oriented coping style; 0.68 for emotion oriented style; 0.75 for task oriented style; 0.59 for the best solution oriented style in the male version and respectively: 0.65; 0.67; 0.71; 0.55 in female version. The validity of the BMECD was assessed with the Polish version of the CISS questionnaire [45] among 125 women and 104 men only. The strongest correlations were found between: found between task-oriented coping style in CISS and combined results for the task oriented and the best-solution oriented coping style in BMECD among women ($r = 0.42$; $p < 0.001$) among men ($r = 0.41$; $p < 0.001$) and between scores in the emotion oriented coping ($r=0.29$; $p < 0.001$ both for men and women). There were no significant correlations between scores in avoidance oriented coping styles in both measures, both in group men and women. Those correlations indicate that the coping styles identified in BMECD have some similarities with those differentiated by CISS, but measure different modes of reaction to stressful events.

The Brief Measure to Assess Perception of Self-Influence on the Disease Course: Version for Diabetes (BMAPS-IDC, published in the appendix)[7]. The BMAPS-IDC questions were developed based on methodology that was discussed during a focus group interview with patients with T2DM who, in the opinion of their doctors, had developed either adaptive or maladaptive styles in order to cope with their disease. This led to the originating of 50 items, each using a 5-point Likert scale to assess outcomes. These 50 items were then modified following a discussion with two persons with diabetes. To further validate the 50-item version of the BMAPS-IDC, the questionnaire was used among 170 patients, in whom their doctor, using clinical judgment, rated the patient's perception of self-influence on the diabetes course.

Statistical analysis (Wald test and logistic regression) identified six items that optimally differentiated the group in terms of high and low perception of self-influence on the disease course; thus, the final BMAPS-IDC questionnaire consisted of six items, each presented using a 5-point Likert scale. Higher BMAPS-IDC scores denote a greater perception of self-influence over the disease course.

The BMAPS-IDC has good reliability (Cronbach's alpha, 0.75) and acceptable validity (Kendall tau, 0.54), as well as a standardized ten scale for the assessment of results, which was created to describe clinically significant differences. According to the ten scale, low raw scores of 0–11 scores correspond with <5 on the ten scale, average raw scores of 12–15 correspond to ten scale scores of 5–6, and high raw scores of 16–24 of translate to 7–10 on the ten scale. There were no meaningful gender differences in scores on this scale. In a study among 655 females and 544 males the mean score in BMAPS-IDC was 14.88 (SD= 4.332) and 14.11 (SD = 4.348) respectively. This difference was statistically significant t = - 3.04, df=1193, p = 0.002, but was not clinically significant [46].

A Brief Self-Rating Scale of Depression and Anxiety (BS-RSDA) [47]. It is a short method for evaluating the intensity of depression and anxiety symptoms, developed with norms for patients with diabetes. It consists of 10 items with an 11 degree Likert scale (from 0 to 10). The overall score therefore falls somewhere between 0 to 100. 5 questions fall in the depression category, 5 into the anxiety one (the result is from 0 to 50 for each of the scales). Construction of these scales was based on most significant psychopathological symptoms characteristic for depression in both classifications – DSM-IV and ICD 10. In the depression scale the following factors were developed: mood, intensity of energy, strength of interests, ability to feel pleasure, speed of thought and action. They constitute elements of depression episode and might appear in other depressive disorders. In case of anxiety there are many categories of anxiety disorders. For the evaluation of anxiety symptoms, the following factors were included: 1. worry, tension, uneasiness; 2. anxiety or fear of specific threat; 3. apprehension, distress; 4. physical tension; 5. desire to avoid situations that cause anxiety.

The tool has good psychometric properties, evaluated on the basis of a study conducted on 240 respondents – patients with diabetes. Both scales proved to have good reliability, the Cronbach's alpha was 0.95 for depression and 0.94 for anxiety. Both scales were also found to be valid. The depression scale correlated with the results of Beck Depression Inventory (r=0.809) and the HADS Depression Scale (r=0.797). The anxiety scale correlated with the results of HADS Anxiety Scale (r=0.805). Reliability of the entire scale was also high (Cronbach's alpha=0.956). Because of the lack of a reference tool, the validity of the whole scale was not measured. High reliability of the subscales was replicated in a study among 101 persons with diabetes: Cronbach's alpha was 0.92 for the depression scale and 0.91 for the anxiety scale. In the study among 133 persons with cardiologic and orthopedic disease in the test-retest reliability measurement, after 30 minutes, the correlation of subscale scores for depression was r=0.845, and for the subscale of anxiety r=0.814

A temporary ten norm scales were developed, and the analysis of relations of the BS-RSDA scores and diagnosis of depression with structured interview indicated that results of depression subscale >11 have sensitivity for detection of depression that is 0.886 and specificity that is 0.727.

2.3. The practical schema of psychotherapeutic management within a regular medical visit [40,44,48]

The schema was created in order to help doctors in making basic psychotherapeutic interventions during the regular visit. Its application was encouraged by series of workshops for doctors treating diabetes in Poland, however it may be used without the training. The main goals of this intervention is helping patients in the stressful problems related with diabetes. The diagnosis focuses on the assessment and practical teaching patients about coping mechanisms, perception of self-influence on the diabetes course and development of patient abilities of problem-solving and use of coping task oriented and "the best solution oriented" coping styles. It eventually broadens the range of behaviors aiming at problem solving. This is congruent with self-management with diabetes based on empowerment. The study [49] shows that a mere transfer of information between the doctor and the patient (regarding the disease and the proposed treatment) does not ensure satisfactory results in terms of the outcome of treatment and the patient's adherence to medical recommendations. An improvement on the doctor-patient relationship has been suggested, basing on the tenets of cognitive behavioral therapy. The traditional model in which the health-care provider is the 'expert' to be consulted by the 'patient' has been replaced by a partnership in which both parties cooperate to achieve best results. In this approach, the patient is the central figure and – acknowledged to be an expert in his/her problematic symptoms - becomes an active member of his/her disease management team. The role of the therapist, on the other hand, is to assist the patient in this process. One of the methods which can be employed by the therapist is the Socratic method in the form of Socratic dialog that enables the patient to determine the problem areas and to guide them to make decisions regarding the course of treatment. Instead of offering ready solutions the therapist is required to guide the patient to work out the solutions to their problems. Thus the patients are empowered to use their own initiative, which shifts the locus of control closer to them and motivates them to effectively manage their own care leading to significant improvements in healthy behavior. In order to achieve this, cognitive behavioral therapy recommends the method of "small steps" whereby the patient is encouraged to make gradual alterations in their habits rather than introduce radical changes. Even modest results serve as positive reinforcement and motivate further efforts. The Schema consists of the following steps:

1.   Welcoming and establishing contact.

– doctor's warm attitude towards the patient

– giving the patient a chance to say what he/she really wants to say

– It is crucial that the doctor establishes good contact with the patient so that the patient feels comfortable enough to confide in the doctor.

2. Discussing the implementation of the last homework.

– realistic estimation of achievements

– realistic estimation of difficulties

When assessing the degree to which the patient succeeded in complying with the doctor's recommendations it is important to ask open questions so as not to exert pressure on the patient or make them feel examined. In order to empower the patient, the doctor needs to appreciate any effort on the part of the patient and analyze any difficulties with which they may be struggling.

3. Setting the goals of the present visit

– asking the patient what he/she would most like to discuss

– in case of problems with making the choices:

• placing the possible goals in order,

• dividing very difficult goals into smaller ones ("step-by-step" approach)

– in case of serious problems in everyday life - adjusting the therapeutic goals to the to this circumstances

The goal which the patient is to pursue, ought to be realistic, specific (clearly defined) and measurable. In establishing the goal, the patient's current problems need to be considered, including non-medical ones, and assess their impact on the illness. If it is needed, the doctor is recommended to suggest taking small steps, which means breaking the goal down into smaller, more achievable goals. This will enhance the chances of success.

4. Medical examination

– adjustment of the set up goals to an outcome of the medical examination and conducting the required diagnostic procedure

The goals need to be established in the context of the patient's general condition. Only after examining the patient appropriate steps can be set.

5. A brief medical psychotherapeutic diagnosis

– screening for depression and anxiety

It may be made with A Brief Self-Rating Scale of Depression and Anxiety or any other diagnostic tool. The patients identified with risk of depressive disorders or anxiety disorders should be referred for a psychiatric consultation.

– dominating style of coping with stress related with the disease

– the feeling of the influence on the course of the disease

The coping style and perception of self-influence on the diabetes course may be made with use of aforementioned. The physician needs to assess how ready the patient is to introduce changes in his/her lifestyle, how strongly he/she believes in the positive outcome of the changes and to what degree the patient feels he/she has the perception of self-influence on a particular problem.

6. Socratic dialog leading to a realistic evaluation of the main problem's source and its possible solutions

– assessment of the problem in the context of general life situation

–formulation of possible solutions

– assessment of advantages and disadvantages of possible solutions

Asking the patient a series of questions enables him/her to determine the source of the problem and to seek the most suitable solution. Since the patient is encouraged to use their own initiative, they will more strongly believe in their ability to achieve their goals.

7. Setting the realistic homework for the period prior to the next visit.

– "small steps" that have good chance for successful outcomes

– defining the criteria of the outcome estimation

– formulating actions that will be taken in case of serious problems with conducting homework

On the basis of the information gathered during the visit, the doctor is recommended to work out a list of recommendations to be implemented by the patient after the visit. It is important to consider any foreseeable difficulties and discuss the means to overcome them.

8. Recapitulation of the visit by the patient

– what are the conclusions of the discussion

– what is the homework to be conducted prior to the following appointment

It is good if the physician asks the patient to recapitulate briefly to make sure that the patient understands the arrangements discussed during the visit

3. Discussion

The Psychodiabetic KIT was created in order to encourage doctors to make psychotherapeutic diagnoses and basic psychotherapeutic interventions that will improve their patients' coping with diabetes. Realistically, it may be helpful during a yearly follow up visit, that according to International Diabetes Federation guidelines [19] should include assessment of psychological functioning of patients with diabetes type 2 or when screening tools or clinical assessment indicate a risk of psychological problems related to diabetes, including comorbid depression or anxiety disorders. The diagnostic tools can be used together or separately. However, it is recommended that the doctor or the nurse using the KIT become familiar with the details of The Brief Method of Evaluating Coping with Disease and are able to use examples of situations and reactions specific for the four main coping styles, in the process of educating the patient about his/her coping styles and, if needed, possibilities of its improvement. It may also be helpful for the patient to get a copy of the questionnaire with the key. It is crucial to explain to the patient that his/her perception of self-influence on the disease course, explain the need for the development by him/her the task oriented coping and the best solution oriented coping for dealing with diabetes related stressful problem. The patients with low level of the perception of self-influence on the disease course need interventions increasing this aspect of illness perception. It includes the "step-by-step" approach to the diabetes related problem together with self-monitoring effects of activity by making written records or self-rating scales. Otherwise, nonadherence to many of therapeutic recommendations among patients with a low perception of self-influence on diabetes course is very likely. Brief Self-Rating Scale of Depression and Anxiety needs specific norms for each language. However, the Polish sten norms can be helpful in a preliminary assessment of the intensity of symptoms of depression and anxiety(detailed ten norms are available from the first author).

They may also be used for the comparison of those symptoms in time. The version of the Psychodiabetic KIT tools included in the Appendix followed the rules of back-translation as it is a commonly accepted methodology in such cases. Still, their psychometric proprieties should be assessed in English speaking countries. Translations into other languages need back-translation procedures and assessment of their psychometric proprieties, before application in research. The main idea of the Psychodiabetic KIT is to facilitate clinical diagnosis, psycho-education of the patient considering coping, perception of self-influence as well as the need for monitoring depression and anxiety. Even non-validated translations of the KIT may be helpful in reaching these goals.

4. Application of the components of psychodiabetic KIT in research

Components of Psychodiabetic KIT were used in several research. This review presents only those which were published, including two cross-sectional, national studies. However, the results of other studies that resulted in on Ph. Thesis, and more than 10 M.A. thesis are currently in process of preparation for publications.

The national, cross- sectional study "Relationship between psychological coping style and insulin pen choice in patients with T2DM" [50] was aiming at assessment of relationship among coping styles and a choice of one of four available pens – insulin injectors that differed in technological complexity, size and accuracy:

- InnoLet – big and disposable, filled with insulin
- NovoLet – small and disposable; filled with insulin
- NovoPen 3 – durable, for multiple use, and filled each time by the patient

Innovo – durable, for multiple use, compact size, that make discretely injection in social situations possible, as well as record of the dosage and time of injection. The study was conducted by general practitioners with subsequent patients and only included a single visit during which treatment with insulin was initiated and when the patient chose an insulin injector. The style of coping was assessed at the same time with the working version of The Brief Method of Evaluating Coping with Disease (BMECD)[24], that had worst psychometric proprieties, assessed on smaller group that final one). The study involved 945 patients (553 females [59.1%]; 382 males [40.9%] – gender data were missing for 10 patients) aged 18–90 years (mean [SD]: 61.7 [11.7] years) who were beginning insulin therapy after a period of treatment for T2DM ranging from several months to 61 years (mean [SD]: 8.3 [5.9] years). The number (proportion) of patients in this study choosing each type of pen was: 460 (48.7%) NovoPen® 3; 269 (28.5%) NovoLet®; 25 (2.6%) Innovo®; 176 (18.6%) InnoLet®; data were missing for 15 (1.6%) patients. Statistically significant differences between mean BMECD scores were found among patients who chose one of four types of insulin pens. The results indicated that an avoidance-oriented coping style was associated with choosing the simplest insulin pen, an emotion-oriented coping style with a more complicated insulin pen, a task-oriented coping style with a modern pen, and the 'the best solution oriented' coping style with the technologically most advanced pen. In spite of many methodological limitations of this study its results encouraged the elaboration of the final version of the BMECD and supported its usefulness in clinical practice.

Another cross-sectional national study [46] involved 480 physicians and 1199 patients (655 females [54.6%]; 544 males [45.4%]) aged 4–93 years (mean [SD]: 62.0 [11.6] years) who were beginning insulin therapy after a period of treatment for diabetes ranging from several months to 36 years (mean [SD]: 8.0 [5.5] years). The study was conducted with consecutive patients and only included a single visit during which treatment with insulin was initiated and when the patient made their choice of insulin injector. Analysis of the relationship between the perception of self-influence on the disease course and choice of insulin pen was possible for 1184 (98.7%) persons enrolled in the study. The Brief Measure to Assess Perception of Self-Influence on the Disease Course: Version for Diabetes (BMAPS-IDC) was applied. The number (proportion) of patients in this study choosing each type of pen was: 538 (44.9%) NovoPen® 3; 383 (31.9%) NovoLet®; 220 (18.4%) InnoLet®; data were missing for 58 (4.8%) patients. In the group that chose the simplest disposable injector – InnoLet® – the mean BMAPS-IDC score (12.23) was significantly lower than in group that chose the smaller and more complicated type of injector (NovoPen® 3, 15.72). The mean BMAPS-IDC score in the group that chose the intermediate injector (NovoLet®, 13.88) lay between, and was statistically different from, the means of the other two groups.

Of the 395 patients in this study with data from relevant assessments, mean HbA_{1c} levels were ≤6.5% (low risk of cardiovascular [CV] complications) in 10 (2.5%) patients; between 6.6 and 7.5% (risk of arterial complications) in 38 (9.6%) patients; and >7.5% in 347 (87.8%) patients. Mean (SD) BMAPS-IDC scores in the groups with low risk of CV complications, risk of arterial complications, and risk of microvascular complications were: 18.20 (2.97), 16.55 (4.38), 14.43 (4.35), respectively. The difference in BMAPS-IDC scores between the group at low risk of CV complications (HbA_{1c} ≤6.5%) and the group at risk of microvascular complications (HbA_{1c} >7.5%) was statistically significant (p<0.01).

A correlation analysis suggested that the perception of self-influence on the course of diabetes has an increasing impact on the effectiveness of the treatment, as assessed by HbA_{1c} levels following long-term treatment. In total, 72 patients had been treated for less than 3 years, 72 for 3 years or more, and 249 for more than 5 years. The correlations were not significant in the group treated for diabetes for less than 3 years. Weak, but statistically significant correlations were found in the group treated for more than 3 years for diabetes (r=-0.18; p<0.05) and for those with a disease length over 5 years (r=-0.2; p<0.05).

Limitations of both of these studies include the observational design, which meant that participating doctors were not blinded to the results and could potentially influence patients' results. Due to the cross-sectional design the data presented in this paper only describe a relationship between coping styles or the perception of self-influence on the disease course and the type of device used at the beginning of insulin therapy, but cannot prove a cause and effect relationship, which may be worthy of further investigation.

Studies, which were presented above, revealed that the coping style and perception of self-influence on the course of diabetes have an important role in the process of the treatment choice. The relationship between the perception of self-influence on the disease course and the effectiveness of the treatment manifested by HbA1c level is also noteworthy.

Overall, the results of these studies indicate that psychological intervention aimed at developing task-oriented and 'the best solution-oriented' coping styles may result in the choice of more precise treatment, allowing more accurate glycemic control. Therefore, helping patients understand and believe that they can control the outcome of their diabetes is of value.

Conversely, clinicians may wish to use these findings to help them identify the coping style and the level of belief in self influence for a particular patient, which could enable further individualization of the treatment plan.

Comparing coping styles, occurrence of depressive and anxiety symptoms, and locus of control among patients with diabetes type 1 and type 2 in groups of 30 with type 1 and 27 with type 2 [51]. In the group of patients with diabetes type 2 there were found significantly higher, than in diabetes type 1: emotion oriented coping style (M = 0.4; SD = 0.814 vs. M = 0.93; SD = 0.958; p = 0.029), avoidance oriented coping style (M = 0.63; SD = 0.809 vs. M = 1.22; SD = 0.892; p = 0.011); level of depression (M = 4.13; SD = 2.662 vs. M = 5.63; SD = 2.911; p = 0.047), attribution of the health control to a chance (M = 19.03; SD = 6.672 vs. M = 24.26; p = 0.004) and also lower task-oriented coping style. (M = 1.8; SD = 1.095 vs. M = 1.07; SD = 0.829; p = 0.007).

What was also found, were the significant relations among the best solution-oriented coping style, emotion oriented style and the level of anxiety (respectively r = - 0.373; r = 0.37) and level of depression (respectively r = - 0.352 i r = 0.476); solution-oriented coping style, emotion-oriented coping style, level of anxiety and with the attribution of the health control to a chance (respectively r = 0.341; r = 0.271; r = 0.301); level of depression and locus of control (r = 0,322), i.e.: higher level of depression is correlated with more external locus of control; attribution of the health control to a chance and the older age (r = 0.407). The results of this preliminary study suggests that patients with diabetes type 2 use more maladaptive coping styles (emotion and avoidance oriented) than patients with diabetes type 1, and that use of specific coping styles is related with depression and anxiety

5. Assessment of psychodiabetic kit by doctors

In a survey conducted during a series of educational conferences in 2006, out of 217 doctors treating patients with diabetes, approximately half of them were acquainted with the BMECD and one-third with the BMAPS-IDC. In addition, 52.6% of doctors familiar with the BMECD, reported using it in everyday practice, and the majority were keen to further develop their experience with psychological tools used for the support of diabetic patients. [52]

6. Conclusions

1. Current guidelines of the International Diabetes Federation [19] and American Diabetes Association [20] as well as consensus statement of the American Diabetes Association and Europeans Association for Study of Diabetes, in respect to current knowledge, recommend individualized patient–centered approach in treatment and management of diabetes type.

2. A team approach, including variety of medical professionals, is recommended by IDF [19] on the "comprehensive" and "recommended" levels of care. However, these guidelines also describe a kind of "limited" care in respect to existence of "settings with very limited resources – drugs, personnel, technologies and procedures" [19].

3. The Psychodiabetic KIT facilitates, brief psychotherapeutic diagnosis and education of patients dealing with coping with diabetes related stressors as well as simply therapeutic interventions based on currently recommended rules of self-management and empowerment aiming at increasing the patients' perception of self-influence on the diabetes course and at the development of task related and "the best solution oriented" coping with stressful problems. It also may be used for depressive disorders and anxiety disorders screening.

4. The results of research indicate that the Brief Method of Evaluating Coping with Disease and the Brief Measure To Assess Perception Of Self- Influence On The Disease Course are useful in research. Their results confirm that coping styles and perception of self-influence on the disease course are related with the choice of treatment modality, i.e. insuline injector. The difference of the level of perception of self- influence on diabetes course was statistically significantly higher in between the group at low risk of CV complications (HbA$_{1c}$ ≤6.5%) than in the group at risk of microvascular complications (HbA$_{1c}$ >7.5%). There were also week, but statistically significant correlations between the perception of self-influence on the course of diabetes, the effectiveness of the treatment, as assessed by HbA$_{1c}$ levels in groups of treated patients. The results of the preliminary study suggest that patients with diabetes type 2 use more maladaptive coping styles (emotion and avoidance oriented) than patients with diabetes type 1, and that a use of specific coping styles is related with depression and anxiety.

5. The results of anonymous survey among Polish doctors treating diabetes indicate that Psychodiabetic KIT may by useful in everyday practice.

Appendix

Brief method of evaluating coping with disease[1]: Version for men (Kokoszka, Radzio, Kot, 2008)

Name……………………………………..Date……………………………..

Please circle one answer to each of the four questions:

1. If you found yourself in a group of people having to deal with a serious problem (among people shamed by a building society authorities or a service company not meeting its obligations), you would most probably:
   a. Do nothing and count on someone else to take care of it or would figure out that its pointless and dealing with it is a waste of time
   b. Look for others who were harmed and, together with them, try to protect my rights
   c. Try to influence the people who got engaged in solving the problem, so that I could get the best outcome
   d. Be mainly angry and upset and would not feel like doing anything

2. When you notice longer-lasting swerves in your health (minor pain, weakness), you usually:
   a. Not worry for a while and wait for them to pass
   b. Worry that it might be a beginning of a serious illness, which may potentially cause problems
   c. Look for information in a health-guide, ask acquaintances who have had similar problems or contact a doctor
   d. Contact a doctor as soon as possible and want to do everything possible to prevent the development of the disorder or at least assuage its course

3. If you had a chance to inherit, but it required a long-drawn participation in a trial, you would probably:
   a. Decline participation as not being sure about the success you wouldn't want to waste time on unpleasant activities
   b. Lodge a lawsuit yourself
   c. Hire a lawyer to best represent your interest
   d. Be irritated by the situation and ask relatives or friends to take care of it

4. When there is a serious conflict between your close-ones, you usually:
   a. Try talking to them in order to resolve the conflict
   b. Do nothing and try to avoid thinking about it
   c. Feel upset and worries because I don't like situations like that
   d. Try to link them to others who had similar problems or talk to them about how others handled similar situations

---

1 The authors gratefully acknowledge permission to translate this method to Via Medica, that published paper: Kokoszka A, Radzio R, Kot W. Krótka Metoda Ocena Radzenia Sobie z Chorobą: wersja dla mężczyzn i kobiet (Brief Method of Evaluating Coping with Disease: versions for men and women). Diabetologia Praktyczna 2008;9(1) 1-11.

Brief method of evaluating coping with disease: Version for women (Kokoszka, Radzio, Kot, 2008)

Name..Date...................................

Please circle one answer to each of the four questions:

1. If you found yourself in a group of people having to deal with a serious problem (with young people disturbing peace in your community, with your superior at work or with the authorities of a building company), you would most probably:

    a. I would try to engage in some other activity and wait patiently, believing that that the problem will be solved

    b. Engage in the activities of the group trying to solve the problem

    c. Try to influence the people who got engaged or lead them myself, but mainly I would try to solve the problem in the best option for me

    d. Be mainly angry and upset and would not feel like doing anything

2. When you notice longer-lasting swerves in your health (minor pain, weakness), you usually:

    a. Hope, they are not serious and wait for them to pass

    b. Worry and are afraid of different possible illnesses

    c. Look for information in a health-guide, ask acquaintances who have had similar problems or contact a doctor

    d. Contact a doctor as soon as possible and want to do everything possible to prevent the development of the disorder or at least assuage its course

3. If you had a chance to inherit, but it required a long-drawn participation in a trial, you would probably:

    a. Resign your participation

    b. Lodge a lawsuit yourself

    c. Hire a lawyer to best represent your interest

    d. Be worried by the need of participating in the procedure and rely on my relatives' opinions

4. When there is a serious, prolonged conflict between your close-ones, you usually:

    a. Try talking to them in order to resolve the conflict

    b. Do nothing and try to avoid thinking about it

    c. Feel upset and worried and want them to solve it as quickly as possible

    d. Try to assess whether they need help and what I could do to offer best possible support

Key for interpreting answers

Versions for both gender

Find each of the patient's answer on the list below then calculate the number of the responses characteristic for each of four coping styles. This result can be discussed with the patient and the answers characteristic for each of the coping style can be used for the patient education on coping styles. In research, row results are used.

Task-oriented coping style

1. b) look for others who were harmed and, together with them, try to protect my rights/ engage in the activities of the group trying to solve the problem
2. c) look for information in a health-guide, ask acquaintances who have had similar problems or contact a doctor
3. b) lodge a lawsuit yourself;
4. a) try talking to them in order to resolve the conflict

Best solution-oriented coping style

1. c) try to influence the people who got engaged in solving the problem, so that I could get the best outcome/ try to influence the people who got engaged or lead them myself, but mainly I would try to solve the problem in the best option for me
2. d) contact a doctor as soon as possible and want to do everything possible to prevent the development of the disorder or at least assuage its course
3. c) hire a lawyer to best represent your interest
4. d) try to link them to others who had similar problems or talk to them about how others handled similar situations/ try to assess whether they need help and what I could do to offer best possible support

Emotion-oriented coping style

1. d) be mainly angry and upset and would not feel like doing anything
2. b) worry that it might be a beginning of a serious illness, which may potentially cause problems/ worry and are afraid of different possible illnesses
3. d) be irritated by the situation and ask relatives or friends to take care of it/ be worried by the need of participating in the procedure and rely on my relatives' opinions
4. c) feel upset and worries because I don't like situations like that/ feel upset and worried and want them to solve it as quickly as possible

Avoidance-oriented coping style

1. a) do nothing and count on someone else to take care of it or would figure out that its pointless and dealing with it is a waste of time/ I would try to engage in some other activity and wait patiently, believing that that the problem will be solved
2. a) not worry for a while and wait for them to pass/ hope, they are not serious and wait for them to pass
3. a) decline participation as not being sure about the success you wouldn't want to waste time on unpleasant activities/ resign your participation
4. b) do nothing and try to avoid thinking about it

The sum of given answers

Task-oriented coping style – ….
Best-solution oriented coping style –....
Emotion-oriented coping style –....
Avoidance-oriented coping style –....

Brief measure to assess perception of self- influence on the disease course (Kokoszka, 2005)[2]

Name...Date...................................

Please circle your personal opinion on each of the following questions:

1. If I take care of myself, I will have a better health

| I fully agree | I rather agree | It is hard to say | I rather disagree | I disagree |

2. If I accomplish all my plans related to the management of diabetes (treatment, diet, physical activity) I generally feel relief

| I fully agree | I rather agree | It is hard to say | I rather disagree | I disagree |

3. I spend a lot of time preventing possible future complications of my illness

| I fully agree | I rather agree | It is hard to say | I rather disagree | I disagree |

4. Diet and lifestyle do not influence my health, because the most important is medication (and insulin)

| I fully agree | I rather agree | It is hard to say | I rather disagree | I disagree |

5. The course of my illness depends mostly on fate

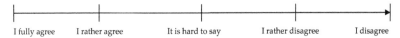

| I fully agree | I rather agree | It is hard to say | I rather disagree | I disagree |

6. The experience gained during therapy helps me to better cope with other problems in my life

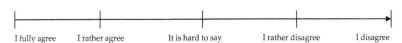

| I fully agree | I rather agree | It is hard to say | I rather disagree | I disagree |

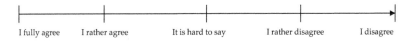

---

2 The authors gratefully acknowledge permission to translate this method to Wydawnictwo Przegląd Lekarski that published the paper: Kokoszka A. Krótka metoda oceny poczucia wpływu na przebieg choroby: opis wersji dla osób z cukrzycą (Brief measure to assess perception of self-influence on the disease course. Version for diabetes).Przegląd Lekarski 2005;62(8) 742-745

Key

Questions 1, 2 ,3, 6	Questions 4, 5 – inverted score
I fully agree – 4	I fully agree – 0
I rather agree – 3	I rather agree – 1
It is hard to say – 2	It is hard to say – 2
I rather disagree –1	I rather disagree – 3
I disagree – 0	I disagree – 4

Interpretation according to standardized ten scale:

Low scores 0-11(< 5 sten)

Average scores 12-15 (5-6 sten)

High scores 16-24 (> 6 sten)

Brief Self- rating scale of depression and anxiety (Kokoszka, 2008) [3]

Name……………………………………..Date………………………………..

Please assess your well-being on the following scales by putting an X in a chosen place of the scale.

You should compare your current well-being with previous feeling of comfort.

Number 10 stands for an intensity of the assessed feature that is the highest that you can imagine.

1. Mood

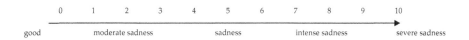

2. Intensity of energy

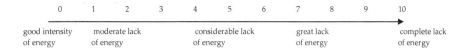

___

3 The authors gratefully acknowledge permission to translate this method to Termedia, that published, the paper: Kokoszka A. Krótka Skala Samooceny Depresji i Lęku: opis konstrukcji oraz właściwości psychometrycznych dla osób z cukrzycą (Brief Self-Rating Scale of Depression and Anxiety: description of the scale construction and psychometric proprieties for persons with diabetes). Przewodnik Lekarza 2008;11(6) 74-81

3. Power of interests

0	1	2	3	4	5	6	7	8	9	10

normal   moderately weakened   considerably weakened   highly weakened   severely weakened

4. The capacity to feel pleasure

0	1	2	3	4	5	6	7	8	9	10

normal   moderately weakened   considerably weakened   highly weakened   severely weakened

5. Speed of thought and action

0	1	2	3	4	5	6	7	8	9	10

normal   moderately weakened   considerably weakened   highly weakened   severely weakened

6. Worry, tenseness, nervousness

0	1	2	3	4	5	6	7	8	9	10

none   moderate   strong   very strong   severe

7. Anxiety (feeling of fear without a certain reason), fear of a specified threat

0	1	2	3	4	5	6	7	8	9	10

none   moderate   strong   very strong   severe

8. Apprehension and distress about something that might happen

0	1	2	3	4	5	6	7	8	9	10

none   moderate   strong   very strong   severe

9. Feeling of physical tension in a body (intense muscle tension, trembling hands, aches)

0	1	2	3	4	5	6	7	8	9	10

none   moderate   strong   very strong   severe

10. Desire to avoid situations that cause anxiety (hiding, withdrawing)

0	1	2	3	4	5	6	7	8	9	10

none   moderate   strong   very strong   severe

Key — Adding the scores 1-5 depression subscale; 6-10 anxiety subscale

Reliability: depression scale α Cronbacha= 0,95; anxiety scale α Cronbacha= 0,94, entire scale α Cronbacha=0,956.

Interpretation according to standardized ten scale:

Depression scale:

Low scores 0-2 (1–4 sten)
Average scores 3-12 (5–6 sten)
High scores 13-50 (7–10 sten)

Anxiety scale:
Low scores 0-4 (1–4 sten)
Average scores 5-14 (5–6sten)
High scores 15-50 (7–10 sten)

Entire scale:
Low scores 0-8 (1–4 sten)
Average scores 9-27 (5–6 sten)
High scores 28-100 (7–10 sten)

Author details

Andrzej Kokoszka[1*], Aleksandra Jodko-Modlińska[2], Marcin Obrębski[2],
Joanna Ostasz-Ważny[1] and Rafał Radzio[2]

*Address all correspondence to: andrzej.kokoszka@wum.edu.pl

1 II Department of Psychiatry, Medical University of Warsaw, Warsaw, Poland

2 University of Social Sciences and Humanities, Warsaw, Poland

References

[1] Inzucchi SE, Bergenstal RM, Buse JB, Diamant M, Ferrannini E, Nauck M, Peters AL, Tsapas A, Wender R, Matthewset DR. American Diabetes Association (ADA)European an Association for the Study of Diabetes (EASD). Management of hyperglycemia in type 2 diabetes: a patient-centered approach. Position statement of the American Diabetes Association (ADA) and the European Association for the Study of Diabetes (EASD). Diabetes Care 2012;35(6) 1364–1379.

[2] Kokoszka A, Sieradzki J. Poczucie wpływu na przebieg choroby a sposób leczenia cukrzycy (Relationship between the feeling of influence on the course of disease and the management with diabetes). Diabetologia Praktyczna 2005;6(1) 1-5.

[3] Kokoszka A, Szmalec M. Relationships of eating disorders with psychological problems in the course of diabetes type 2: cross-sectional study. The 14th Scientific Meeting of the PSAD Psycho Social Aspects of Diabetes Study (PSAD) Group at the European Association for the Study of Diabetes, Dubrovnik, 2009.

[4] Ali S, Stone MA, Peters JL, Davies MJ, Khunti K. The prevalence of co-morbid depression in adults with Type 2 diabetes: a systematic review and meta-analysis. Diabetic Medicine 2006;23(11) 1165-1173.

[5] Cuijpers P, Smith F. Subthreshold depression is a risk factor for major depressive disorder. A systematic review of prospective studies. Acta Psychiatrica Scandinavica 2004;109(5) 325-331.

[6] Kokoszka A, Radzio R, Kot W. Krótka Metoda Oceny Radzenia Sobie z Chorobą: wersja dla mężczyzn i kobiet (Brief Method of Evaluating Coping with Disease: versions for men and women). Diabetologia Praktyczna 2008;9(1) 1-11.

[7] Kokoszka A. Krótka metoda oceny poczucia wpływu na przebieg choroby: opis wersji dla osób z cukrzycą (Brief measure to assess perception of self-influence on the disease course. Version for diabetes). Przegląd Lekarski 2005;62(8) 742-745.

[8] Zulman DM, Rosland AM, Choi H, Langa KM, Heisler M. The influence of diabetes psychosocial attributes and self-management practices on change in diabetes status. Patient Education And Counseling 2012;87(1) 74-80.

[9] King DK, Glasgow RE, Toobert DJ, Strycker LA, Estabrooks PA, Osuna D, Faber AJ. Self-efficacy, problem solving, and social-environmental support are associated with diabetes self-management behaviors. Diabetes Care 2010;33(4) 751-753.

[10] Greenfield C, Gilles M, Porter C, Shaw P, Willis K. It's not just about the HbA1c, Doc! Understanding the psychosocial is also important in managing diabetes? The Australian Journal Of Rural Health 2011;19(1) 15-19.

[11] Peyrot M, Rubin RR, Lauritzen T, Snoek FJ, Matthews DR, Skovlund SE. Psychosocial problems and barriers to improved diabetes management: results of the Cross-National Diabetes Attitudes, Wishes and Needs (DAWN) Study. Diabetic Medicine 2005;22(10) 1379-1385.

[12] Snoek FJ, Kersch NYA, Eldrup E, Harman-Boehm I, Hermanns N, Kokoszka A, Matthews DR, McGuire BE, Pibernik-Okanovic M, Singer J, de Wit M, Skovlund SE. Monitoring of Individual Needs in Diabetes (MIND)-2: Follow-up data from the cross-national Diabetes Attitudes, Wishes, and Needs (DAWN) MIND study. Diabetes Care 2012;35(11) 2128-2132.

[13] Snoek FJ, Kersch NYA, Eldrup E, Harman-Boehm I, Hermanns N, Kokoszka A, Mat-
      thews DR, McGuire BE, Pibernik-Okanovic M, Singer J, de Wit M, Skovlund SE.
      Monitoring of Individual Needs in Diabetes (MIND): baseline data from the Cross-
      National Diabetes Attitudes, Wishes, and Needs (DAWN) MIND study. Diabetes
      Care 2011;34(3) 601–603.

[14] Bech P, Olsen RL, Kjoller M, Rasmussen NK. Measuring well-being rather than the
      absence of distress symptoms: a comparison of the SF-36 Mental Health subscale and
      the WHO-Five Well-Being Scale. International Journal Of Methods In Psychiatric Re-
      search 2003;12(2) 85-91.

[15] Bech P. Measuring the dimensions of psychological general well-being by the
      WHO-5. Quality of Life Newsletter 2004;32 15-16.

[16] Snoek FJ, Pouwer F, Welch G, Polonsky WH. Diabetes- related emotional distress in
      Dutch and U.S. diabetic patients. Cross- cultural validity of the Problem Areas in
      Diabetes Scale (PAID). Diabetes Care 2000;23(9) 1305-1309.

[17] Welch GW, Jacobson AM, Polonsky WH. The problem areas in diabetes scale. An
      evaluation of its clinical utility. Diabetes Care 1997;20(5) 760-766.

[18] Polonsky WH, Anderson BJ, Lohrer PA, Welch G, Jacobson AM, Aponte JE, Schwartz
      CE: Assessment of diabetes- related distress. Diabetes care 1995;18(6) 754-760.

[19] International Diabetes Federation, Global Guideline for Type 2 Diabetes, Internation-
      al Diabetes Federation. Brussels, 2012.

[20] Standards of Medical Care in Diabetes—2011. Diabetes Care 2011;34(Suppl. 1) 11-61.

[21] Lazarus RS. Folkman S. Stress, Appraisal and Coping. New York: Springer; 1984.

[22] Tuncay T, Musabak I, Gok DE, Kutlu M. The relationship between anxiety, coping
      strategies and characteristics of patients with diabetes. Health and Quality of Life
      Outcomes 2008;6:79 http://www.hqlo.com/content/6/1/79 (accessed 13 October 2008).

[23] Endler N.S., Parkeri.D"A.: Multidimensional assessment of coping: A critical evalua-
      tion. Journal Of Personality And Social Psychology1990;58(5) 844-854.

[24] Kokoszka A, Jodko A, Radzio R. Krótka metoda radzenia sobie z chorobą – geneza i
      opis roboczej wersji metody [Brief Method of Evaluating Coping with Disease – de-
      scription of the preliminary version]. Przewodnik Lekarza 2003;6(10) 39–46.

[25] Selye H. Stress of life. New York: McGraw-Hill; 1956.

[26] Selye H. Stress in health and disease. Massachusetts: Butterworth's Reading; 1976.

[27] Everly GS, Rosenfeld R. The Nature and Treatment of the Stress Response. New
      York: Plenum; 1981.

[28] Bandura A. Self-efficacy. In: Ramachaudran V.S. (ed.) Encyclopedia of Human Behavior, Vol. 4. New York: Academic Press 1994. p71–81.

[29] Conway VJ, Terry DJ. Appraised controllability as a moderator of the effectiveness of different coping strategies: A test of the goodness of fit hypothesis. Australian Journal of Psychology 1992;44(1) 1–7.

[30] Macrodimitris SD, Endler NS. Coping, control and adjustment in type 2 diabetes. Health Psychology 2001;20(3) 208–216.

[31] Rubin RR, Peyrot M. Quality of life and diabetes. Diabetes/Metabolism Research And Reviews 1999;15(3) 205–218.

[32] Watkins KW, Connell CM, Fitzgerald JT, Klem L, Hickey T, Ingersoll-Dayton B. Effect of adults' self-regulation of diabetes on quality-of-life outcomes. Diabetes Care 2000;23(10) 1511–1515.

[33] Anderson RJ, Freedland KE, Clouse RE, Lustman PJ. The prevalence of comorbid depression in adults with diabetes: a meta-analysis. Diabetes Care 2001;24(6) 1069-1078.

[34] Lustman PJ, Anderson RJ, Freedland KE, de Groot M, Carney RM, Clouse RE. Depression and poor glycemic control: a meta-analytic review of the literature. Diabetes Care 2000;23(7) 934-942.

[35] Katon WJ, Rutter C, Simon G, Lin EH, Ludman E, Ciechanowski P, Kinder L, Young B, Von Korff M. The association of comorbid depression with mortality in patients with type 2 diabetes. Diabetes Care 2005;28(11) 2668-2672.

[36] Beverly EA, Ganda OP, Ritholz MD, Lee Y, Brooks KM, Lewis-Schroeder NF, Hirose M, Weinger K. Look who's (not) talking: diabetic patients' willingness to discuss self-care with physicians. Diabetes Care 2012;35(7) 1466-1472.

[37] Fisher L, Skaff MM, Mullan JT, Arean P, Glasgow R, Masharani U. A longitudinal study of affective and anxiety disorders, depressive affect and diabetes distress in adults with Type 2 diabetes. Diabetic Medicine 2008;25(9) 1096-1101.

[38] Collins MM, Corcoran P, Perry IJ. Anxiety and depression symptoms in patients with diabetes. Diabetes Care 2009;26(2) 153-161.

[39] Lewko J, Zarzycki W, Krajewska-Kulak E. Relationship between the occurrence of symptoms of anxiety and depression, quality of life, and level of acceptance of illness in patients with type 2 diabetes. Saudi Medical Journal 2012;33(8) 887-894.

[40] Kokoszka A, Santorski J. Psychodiabetologia dla lekarzy: postępowanie psychoterapeutyczne w cukrzycy (Psychodiabetology for physicians. Psychotherapeutic management in diabetes). Warszawa: Marketing and Media; 2003.

[41] Kokoszka A. Psychodiabetologia dla lekarzy. Część II: Ocena i kształtowanie poczucia wpływu na przebieg choroby u osób z cukrzycą (Psychodiabetology for physi-

cians. Part II: The assessment and shaping of perception of an influence on the course of disease in diabetes). Warszawa: Pracownia; 2005.

[42] Kokoszka A. Psychodiabetologia dla lekarzy. Cześć III: Zaburzenia depresyjne w przebiegu cukrzycy (Psychodiabetology for physicians. Part III: Depressive disorders in the course of diabetes). Warszawa: Medical Communications; 2007.

[43] Kokoszka A. Psychodiabetologia dla lekarzy. Część IV. Zaburzenia depresyjne i lęk w cukrzycy: Postępowanie w praktyce klinicznej (Psychodiabetology for physicians. Part IV: Anxiety and Depression in clinical practice). Warszawa: Medical Communications; 2010.

[44] Kokoszka A. Diagnoza i postępowanie psychoterapeutyczne w cukrzycy: Zestaw Psychodiabetologiczny (Psychotherapeutic diagnosis and management in diabetes: Psycho-Diabetic Kit). Psychiatria w Praktyce Ogólnolekarskiej 2005;5(4) 146-152.

[45] Endler NS, Parker JDA. Assessment of multidimensional coping: Task, emotion and avoidance strategies. Psychological Assessment 1994;6(1) 50–60.

[46] Kokoszka A, Sieradzki J. Poczucie wpływu na przebieg choroby a sposób leczenia cukrzycy (Relationship between the feeling of influence on the course of disease and the management with diabetes). Diabetologia Praktyczna 2005;6(1) 1–5.

[47] Kokoszka A. Krótka Skala Samooceny Depresji i Lęku: opis konstrukcji oraz właściwości psychometrycznych dla osób z cukrzycą (Brief Self-Rating Scale of Depression and Anxiety: description of the scale construction and psychometric proprieties for persons with diabetes). Przewodnik Lekarza 2008;11(6) 74-81.

[48] Kokoszka A. Schemat psychoterapeutycznej diagnozy i interwencji psychoterapeutycznych w praktyce ogólnolekarskiej (Schema of psychotherapeutic diagnosis and of psychotherapeutic interventions in general medical practice). Przewodnik Lekarza 2004;7(5) 60–69.

[49] Anderson R., Funnell M., Carlson A., Saleh-Statin N., Cradock S., Skinner T.C. Facilitating self-care through empowerment. In: Snoek FJ, Skinner TC (ed.) Psychology in Diabetes Care. Chichester: John Wiley & Sons; 2000. p69–97.

[50] Kokoszka A, Sieradzki J. Styl radzenia sobie z chorobą a wybór rodzaju wstrzykiwacza insuliny u chorych na cukrzycę typu 2 rozpoczynających insulinoterapię (The relationship of style of coping and choice of pen type at the beginning of insulinotherapy in type 2 diabetes). Diabetologia Praktyczna 2004;5(2) 67–74.

[51] Mućko P, Kokoszka A, Skłodowska Z. Porównanie stylów radzenia sobie z chorobą, występowania objawów depresyjnych i lękowych oraz lokalizacji poczucia kontroli u chorych na cukrzycę typu 1 i 2 (The comparison of coping styles, occurrence of depressive and anxiety symptoms, and locus of control among patients with diabetes type 1 and type 2). Diabetologia Praktyczna 2005;6 (5) 240-246.

[52] Kot W, Kokoszka A, Sieradzki J. Ocena zestawu psychodiabetolgicznego oraz potrzeb szkoleniowych z psychodiabetologii wśród lekarzy zajmujących się leczeniem cukrzycy (Assessment of psychodiabetologic kit and psychodiabetology training needs of doctors treating patients with diabetes). Diabetologia Praktyczna 2006;7(6) 405–408.

Permissions

The contributors of this book come from diverse backgrounds, making this book a truly international effort. This book will bring forth new frontiers with its revolutionizing research information and detailed analysis of the nascent developments around the world.

We would like to thank Associate Professor Kazuko Masuo, MD, PhD, for lending his expertise to make the book truly unique. He has played a crucial role in the development of this book. Without his invaluable contribution this book wouldn't have been possible. He has made vital efforts to compile up to date information on the varied aspects of this subject to make this book a valuable addition to the collection of many professionals and students.

This book was conceptualized with the vision of imparting up-to-date information and advanced data in this field. To ensure the same, a matchless editorial board was set up. Every individual on the board went through rigorous rounds of assessment to prove their worth. After which they invested a large part of their time researching and compiling the most relevant data for our readers. Conferences and sessions were held from time to time between the editorial board and the contributing authors to present the data in the most comprehensible form. The editorial team has worked tirelessly to provide valuable and valid information to help people across the globe.

Every chapter published in this book has been scrutinized by our experts. Their significance has been extensively debated. The topics covered herein carry significant findings which will fuel the growth of the discipline. They may even be implemented as practical applications or may be referred to as a beginning point for another development. Chapters in this book were first published by InTech; hereby published with permission under the Creative Commons Attribution License or equivalent.

The editorial board has been involved in producing this book since its inception. They have spent rigorous hours researching and exploring the diverse topics which have resulted in the successful publishing of this book. They have passed on their knowledge of decades through this book. To expedite this challenging task, the publisher supported the team at every step. A small team of assistant editors was also appointed to further simplify the editing procedure and attain best results for the readers.

Our editorial team has been hand-picked from every corner of the world. Their multi-ethnicity adds dynamic inputs to the discussions which result in innovative outcomes. These outcomes are then further discussed with the researchers and contributors who give their valuable feedback and opinion regarding the same. The feedback is then collaborated with the researches and they are edited in a comprehensive manner to aid the understanding of the subject.

Apart from the editorial board, the designing team has also invested a significant amount of their time in understanding the subject and creating the most relevant covers. They scrutinized every image to scout for the most suitable representation of the subject and create an appropriate cover for the book.

The publishing team has been involved in this book since its early stages. They were actively engaged in every process, be it collecting the data, connecting with the contributors or procuring relevant information. The team has been an ardent support to the editorial, designing and production team. Their endless efforts to recruit the best for this project, has resulted in the accomplishment of this book. They are a veteran in the field of academics and their pool of knowledge is as vast as their experience in printing. Their expertise and guidance has proved useful at every step. Their uncompromising quality standards have made this book an exceptional effort. Their encouragement from time to time has been an inspiration for everyone.

The publisher and the editorial board hope that this book will prove to be a valuable piece of knowledge for researchers, students, practitioners and scholars across the globe.

List of Contributors

Gina Agarwal
Department of Family Medicine, McMaster University, Canada

Kazuko Masuo
Nucleus Network Ltd., Baker IDI Heart & Diabetes Institute, Australia
Human Neurotransmitters Laboratory, Baker IDI Heart & Diabetes Institute, Australia

Rashid M. Ansari, John B. Dixon and Colette J. Browning
School of Primary Health Care, Faculty of Medicine, Nursing and Health Sciences, Monash University, Notting Hill, Australia

Daniela Seelenfreund, Nicolas Palou, Sergio Lobos and Rodrigo González
Department of Biochemistry, Faculty of Chemical and Pharmaceutical Sciences, University of Chile, Providencia, Santiago, Chile

Pilar Durruty
Diabetes Unit, Department of Medicine, Faculty of Medicine, University of Chile, Santiago, Chile

Roberto Pontarolo, Astrid Wiens, Helena Hiemisch Lobo Borba, Luana Lenzi and Suelem Tavares da Silva Penteado
Department of Pharmacy – Federal University of Paraná, Curitiba, Paraná, Brazil

Andréia Cristina Conegero Sanches
Department of Medical and Pharmaceutical Sciences - State University of West of Paraná, Cascavel, Paraná, Brazil

Shara S. Azad and Shaker A. Mousa
Pharmaceutical Research Institute, Albany College of Pharmacy and Health Sciences, 1 Discovery Drive, Rensselaer, NY, USA

Esma R. Isenovic
Vinca Institute, University of Belgrade, Department for Molecular Genetics and Radiobiology, Belgrade, Serbia

Subhashini Yaturu
Stratton Veterans Affairs Medical Center / Albany Medical College, Albany, NY, USA

Raymond G. Lau and Collin E. Brathwaite
Department of Bariatric Surgery, Winthrop University Hospital, Mineola, New York, USA

Michael Radin
Department of Endocrinology and Metabolism, Winthrop University Hospital, Mineola, New York, USA

Louis Ragolia
Department of Vascular Biology, Winthrop University Hospital, Mineola, New York, USA

Naruemon Leelayuwat
Department of Physiology, Faculty of Medicine, Khon Kaen University, Thailand

Andrzej Kokoszka and Joanna Ostasz-Ważny
II Department of Psychiatry, Medical University of Warsaw, Warsaw, Poland

Aleksandra Jodko-Modlińska, Marcin Obrębski and Rafał Radzio
University of Social Sciences and Humanities, Warsaw, Poland